Health Informatics and Program Creation

HEALTH INFORMATICS AND PROGRAM CREATION

Taking Action Beyond the Electronic Health Record

FREIDA PEMBERTON

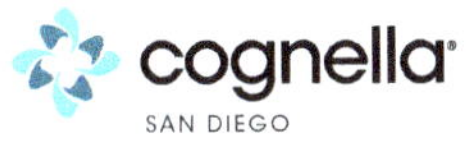

Bassim Hamadeh, CEO and Publisher
Amanda Martin, Executive Publisher
Amy Smith, Associate Editorial Manager
Susana Christie, Senior Developmental Editor
Rachel Kahn, Production Editor
Jess Estrella, Senior Graphic Designer
Karisa Kampbell, Licensing Coordinator
Natalie Piccotti, Director of Marketing
Kassie Graves, Senior Vice President, Editorial
Alia Bales, Director, Project Editorial and Production

Printed in the United States of America.

Brief Contents

Detailed Contents

Preface

The primary objective of this book is to inspire and empower readers like you, aspiring creators who aim to design innovative tools in digital health using programs and advancements in technology. Inspired by modern problems across a wide range of health care needs set against diverse contemporary environments, we embark on the intriguing learning journey that takes us through concept mapping at scale before synthesizing all prior course content within more sophisticated algorithms implemented within groundbreaking solutions for well-being.

Purpose

Central to your success is mastering communication principles, data analytics, information technology, algorithms, advancements in artificial intelligence, core informatics principles, digital health models, leadership and management in informatics. By leveraging Bloom's taxonomy and algorithmic frameworks, this book illuminates the path to developing transformative digital health programs, complete with detailed modeling instructions. Informatics students often struggle to grasp the big picture, focusing narrowly on specific applications without understanding their underlying concepts. As future informaticists, it's crucial to navigate complex manuals and varied vendor product solutions with ease. This book emphasizes the importance of conceptual understanding, helping you innovatively bridge health and technology to address broader societal needs.

Prepare to connect theories, concepts, and informatics models through the integration of digital platforms with health systems beyond the electronic health record (EHR). The unique programs highlighted in this book reflect the assimilation of health informatics principles, aimed at improving and sustaining healthy lifestyle behaviors for individuals, families, and communities. These initiatives empower patients to become effective self-managers of care, fostering projects that allow caregivers and patients to focus on restoring, maintaining, and integrating healthier practices tailored to individual needs.

By the end of this book, you will possess not only the technical skills, but also the conceptual insights necessary to create impactful digital health programs. This book aims to empower you to navigate the digital health care landscape confidently and make meaningful contributions to the field.

Audience

This book is for nursing informatics students, health care informatics students and health care professionals, educators, and administrators who are eager to deepen their understanding of technology's role in health care. Whether you are a student looking to build a strong foundation, an educator seeking to enrich your curriculum, or a professional aiming to stay ahead in your field, this book provides the essential knowledge and skills you need. The goal is to empower you to harness technology effectively and make a significant impact in health care.

Those interested in expanding their understanding of the evolving role of information technology and communication networks in modern health care systems will find this resource beneficial. At its essence, this publication offers the necessary knowledge to address these aspects, empowering everyone. Health care informatics is a major specialty that consistently engages specialists to create technology that better communicates and manages data, transitioning it to information, knowledge, and wisdom. It extends far beyond the EHR to provide quality, tailored health care to a global population.

This textbook is for those who believe that understanding technology's role and contribution deepens both their knowledge and commitment to its use. It suits graduate health informatics students wanting a solid base, educators aiming to enhance their curriculum, and health care professionals seeking to stay ahead.

It offers essential knowledge and skills to harness technology effectively, helping you navigate complex challenges in today's evolving, technology-driven landscape. Experts manage data, transform it into information, and use data analysis to make knowledge applicable to real-life challenges.

Features and Benefits

This book illustrates instructional strategies for engaging students in creating innovative telehealth programs. Key features include these:

- Concept connection charts: These charts link various processes (e.g., problem solving, research, nursing, and algorithms) to enhance understanding.
- Uniform resource locators (URLs): Links to additional readings and original works demonstrate the analysis process and means-end findings.
- Keywords and focus points: Each chapter includes lists of keywords, objectives that lead to outcomes, and focus points to help identify and address knowledge gaps.
- Case scenarios: Thought-provoking scenarios at the end of each unit with multiple-choice questions to encourage practical application.
- Guided assignments: Various assignments show the effectiveness of modeling instructions and demonstrate the culmination of knowledge in computer, information, and telecommunication sciences across health-related fields.
- Visuals: Each chapter includes visuals such as website pages, concept maps, case studies, charts, and images to support understanding, critical thinking, and content transition.
- Original telehealth programs: The text features programs like "The Health Guardian for Longevity Program," for incorporating humor to illustrate meaningful technology use.

The book progresses beyond EHR management, offering opportunities to brainstorm and create solutions for societal health care needs, including those without insurance. It is particularly beneficial for graduate nursing and health informatics students in capstone courses, bridging prior learning to advanced application and preparation for certifications. The final chapter explores career opportunities, including consultant, entrepreneur, project manager, project analyst, application specialist, chief informatics officer, and researcher.

Acknowledgments

This book truly wouldn't exist without the unwavering support and encouragement from my adult children and family. Their early embrace of technology and its integration into our lives has been a constant source of inspiration. To my students, thank you for your enthusiasm and support over the past 51 years, which drove me to move beyond article publications and take on this book. Thus, I dedicate this book to Lashanda Stone, MSW, daughter; Ronald Rhea Jr., BS, son; Cheriese Pemberton, MA, MS, EdD, daughter; and Maya Lucille Stone, granddaughter.

I also want to extend a heartfelt thank you to the incredible Cognella Academic Publishing team: Amanda Martin, executive publisher, nursing and health sciences; Amy Smith, associate editorial manager; Susana Christie, senior developmental editor; and Jess Estrella, senior graphic designer. Your guidance and dedication to this project have been exceptional and vital in bringing this book to life.

Reviewers

Celeste M. Baldwin, PhD, MS, APRN, CNS, GAHN
Assistant Professor for the Online DNP Program
Regis College
Young School of Nursing

Victoria Mills, MBA, RHIA
Gordon State College

Barbara Pinekenstein, DNP, NI-RN, CPHIMS, FAAN
HC Leaders, LLC

Tiffiny Shockley, PhD, MBA, CPHIMS, CHTS-CP, CPEHR
Queens University of Charlotte

Chapter 1

Using Technology to Reinforce

A Guide to Creating Databases

Introduction

The purpose of this chapter is to explore the strategic integration of technology in health care to tackle pressing health issues. It begins by identifying critical health care dilemmas for which technological advancements offer transformative potential. Subsequently, it delves into an in-depth examination of foundational components such as research methodologies, the nursing process, and algorithmic frameworks. Moreover, it scrutinizes the intricate realm of data management, emphasizing the systematic aggregation and comprehension of complex database structures. Through this comprehensive exploration, the chapter aims to equip readers with the knowledge and skills necessary to harness technology effectively in addressing contemporary health care challenges.

This chapter underscores the paramount importance of leveraging technology to enhance health care delivery and outcomes. By providing a nuanced understanding of research principles, clinical methodologies, and data management strategies, it empowers health care professionals to navigate the dynamic landscape of modern health care effectively. Moreover, by fostering proficiency in technological integration, the chapter seeks to optimize patient care, improve health care accessibility, and address the evolving needs of societies on a global scale. In essence, it endeavors to bridge the gap between technological innovation and health care practice, ultimately striving toward a more efficient, equitable, and patient-centric health care system.

The beginning refresher chapters will begin with the identification of a health issue or a crisis that would benefit from the meaningful use of technology. Consider this scenario: a health-related conundrum, wherein strategic technological utilization could yield transformative outcomes. Be it augmenting health care accessibility or optimizing patient data management, our aim is to navigate you through the intricacies of employing technology meaningfully to address these pertinent challenges.

To initiate our discourse, we will embark on a foundational exploration encompassing research principles, the nursing process, and algorithms—the quintessential components underpinning scientific problem solving. Subsequently, we will scrutinize the realm of data—its systematic aggregation, comprehension of intricate database structures, and adept utilization to realize our objectives.

A process will be identified to move the thought forward, starting with research principles, nursing process, and the algorithm process, all under the umbrella of the scientific problem-solving process. The capture of data will be modeled, so that readers understand database tables and how to use them. Following the applications will lead to meaningful use of technology to address the health care needs of society worldwide.

In Chapter 1, our aim is to guide graduate-level health informatics students in leveraging their advanced expertise to integrate database management principles into the initial phases of developing health-related programs. We provide a structured approach, delineating key steps from identifying data sources to designing database schemas, enabling students to apply their knowledge effectively in real-world settings.

Objectives That Lead to Outcomes

We have outlined the specific objectives and expected outcomes for this chapter. The following table aligns key objectives with their corresponding outcomes, providing a clear and detailed understanding of what learners should achieve and comprehend upon completion. This alignment ensures that each objective is met with a tangible and measurable outcome, enhancing the overall learning experience.

Objective	Outcome
Define and explain the relevance of a system in the context of computer and health care information systems (HCIS).	Comprehend the concept of a system and its critical importance in both computer and HCIS, recognizing how systems theory applies to these contexts.
Provide an overview of the basic components of a computer system (hardware, software, data) and their interrelations.	Gain comprehensive knowledge of the fundamental components of a computer system—hardware, software, and data—and how these components interact and depend on each other for optimal functioning.
Define *health care information system* and discuss its types, functions, and benefits in health care.	Attain a thorough understanding of HCIS, including various types (such as electronic health records, radiology information systems, and laboratory information systems), their specific functions, and the benefits they provide to health care organizations and patient care.
Explain the significance of data handling/management in health care, differentiating between structured and unstructured data.	Acquire insight into the critical role of data handling and management in health care, understanding the differences between structured and unstructured data and appreciating the unique value and challenges each type presents in clinical settings.
Introduce tools and techniques for managing health care data, including database management systems (DBMS) and data analytics.	Demonstrate proficiency with various tools and techniques for effectively managing health care data, such as DBMS and data analytics, and how these tools enhance data integrity, accessibility, and utilization in health care.

Objective	Outcome
Emphasize the importance of interoperability and integration between different health care system applications to enhance health care delivery.	Recognize the essential need for interoperability and integration among different health care system applications, understanding how seamless communication and data exchange between systems can significantly improve health care delivery and patient outcomes.

Key Terms

Directions: Before reading, please look at this list of key terms that will be used in this chapter. If any term is unfamiliar, please see the glossary at the end of the book.

computer system
configuration
data
data analysis
data elements
data sources
database management
database schemas
hardware
health
health care information systems
health-related program
information management
interoperability
software
structured data
system
unstructured data

Chapter 1 will provide an introduction related to the history of the generation of computers, providing a context for the presentation on health care information systems (HCIS). Understanding the evolution of computer technology and its impact on health care provides a foundation for discussions on the current state and future direction of HCIS computer systems, and data management that will be required when progressing from theory knowledge acquirement to the development of a product designed to address a societal need. As an informatics specialist, understanding the interplay among system, computer systems, HCIS, interoperability, integration, and data management is crucial. These components work together to create a cohesive, efficient, and effective health care system. By mastering these concepts, informatics specialists can help health care organizations leverage technology to provide better care, improve patient outcomes, and drive down costs. Overall, this understanding is essential for anyone working in nursing and health care informatics.

Integrating Technology in Health Care Program Development

Understanding Systems in Health Care

Integrating computers into the field of health care has been a gradual process marked by the sustained interest and involvement of various health care professionals. While it may be challenging to pinpoint an exact starting point, we can trace several significant milestones that have contributed to the use of computers in health care.

One of the earliest applications of computers in health care occurred during the 1950s and 1960s, when medical researchers began using computers to help analyze and process large volumes of data. This involved leveraging the computing power of machines to conduct complex analyses that would have been difficult, if not impossible, to accomplish by hand.

An essential development during this period was the creation of the Medical Literature Analysis and Retrieval System (MEDLARS) database by the National Library of Medicine. This groundbreaking initiative, launched in 1965, allowed researchers to search and access medical literature electronically, marking a significant shift from traditional manual information retrieval methods (Dee, 2007). With MEDLARS, researchers could access a vast array of medical literature with greater speed and efficiency, ultimately enhancing the quality and depth of health care research.

In the 1970s, the development of electronic health records (EHRs) began to gain traction, particularly in the United States. One of the earliest known EHR systems was developed by a hospital informatics team to improve clinical documentation and decision-making. Around the same time, a research institute affiliated with a health system created one of the first system-wide EHRs, aiming to enhance patient data accessibility across multiple facilities. Initially, these systems were primarily used for billing and administrative functions, but their capabilities expanded in the following decades.

By the 1980s and 1990s, health care informatics emerged as a field of study focused on improving health care through information technology. This led to the development of new applications and systems, such as clinical decision support tools and electronic prescribing systems, designed by physicians and other clinical providers to enhance patient care. Nurses, pharmacists, and other health professionals also played key roles in advancing and implementing these technologies (Reznick, 2017).

As these technological advancements continue to shape modern health care, effective instructional models are essential in preparing professionals to navigate and innovate within this evolving landscape. Gagne's model of instructional design provides an organizational framework to progress from conceptual comprehension of core content to the development of innovative technological, management, and information systems tailored to the health challenges of a global society (Gagne, 1985). Through this framework, professionals gain an understanding of how these systems function and integrate within the broader healthcare landscape.

With the evolution of health care technology, the interconnection among system operation, computer operation, and database management has become increasingly evident. These components are essential to modern computing, ensuring efficient and secure information processing, storage, and access.

Health care technology has now entered its fifth generation, marking the rise of artificial intelligence (AI) and further integrating these systems. Emerging innovations and refinements to existing technologies will continue to strengthen their synergy, enhancing patient care and outcomes. The early adoption of computers in health care marked the beginning of a transformative shift—one that continues to drive innovation today.

System Overview

Components of a Computer System

A system is a structured arrangement of components, processes, and functions designed to achieve a specific purpose. It operates through defined mechanisms that govern its functionality, security, and usability. A complete system includes essential elements such as installation procedures, security protocols, usage instructions, and links to relevant documentation or support resources. Legal notices and terms of service should also be incorporated where necessary.

To ensure effective implementation, it is important to answer questions such as what the outcome is, what the plan is, who will be responsible, and who will be involved. The coordination of activities and consultation with relevant parties must also be considered. Finally, the effectiveness of the solution must be evaluated.

In this specialty, it's important to be familiar with theories related to change and information processing, such as the Kurt Lewin's change theory. Lewin's freeze and refreeze change theory is effective in bringing about change, as opposed to keeping the status quo. Lewin refers to the change model as a method to influence change, getting stakeholders to buy in and embrace the advancements in technology. This theory can help inform informatics health care providers in decision-making and problem-solving processes when integrating new technologies and processes in health care throughout the life cycle.

The use and maintenance of computer systems, networks, and infrastructure involves a set of tasks known as system operation. This encompasses various activities, such as hardware and software installation, network configuration, system performance monitoring, and troubleshooting issues that arise. Computer operation involves the management and use of individual computers and tasks, such as operating system management, software installation and configuration, user management, and device maintenance.

Data Handling and Management in Health Care

Data management is another essential aspect of computing that involves organizing, storing, and manipulating data. It encompasses various tasks, such as data entry, data cleansing, data storage and retrieval, database management, and data analysis. Information management involves the collection, analysis, and dissemination of information to support decision-making and achieve business objectives. This includes tasks such as information governance, information security, data warehousing, and business intelligence.

The transition from system operation to computer operation, to data management, to information management involves increasing levels of complexity and responsibility, as well as a greater focus on using data and information to achieve strategic goals. Therefore, mastering each of these aspects of computing is essential for organizations to stay competitive in today's digital landscape.

Overview of Computer System

A computer system sophisticatedly combines various electronic devices and components that work together to accomplish specific tasks. These components can be broadly classified into three main categories: hardware, software, and data.

Hardware refers to the physical components of a computer system, including the central processing unit (CPU), memory, storage devices, input/output devices, and peripherals such as scanners and webcams. The CPU, also known as the brain of the computer, performs all the processing and calculations. The random access memory (RAM) is used for temporary data storage, while the read-only memory (ROM) is used for permanent data storage on devices like hard drives and solid-state drives.

Software is a collection of programs and applications that run on the computer system. It includes the operating system, such as Windows, MacOS, or Linux; productivity software like word processors and spreadsheets; graphics and design software; and a range of other applications that assist with various tasks.

Data is the information that is processed, stored, and communicated by the computer system. It includes various types of data, such as documents, images, videos, audio files, and other forms of data. Together, hardware, software, and data make up the key components of a computer system that enable it to perform the tasks it was designed to do.

Overall, a computer system is made up of hardware components that process and store data; software that runs on the system and manages its resources; and data that is processed, stored, and communicated by the system. All these components work together to form a complete computer system that can perform a wide range of tasks, from basic functions such as word processing and web browsing to complex tasks such as scientific simulations and data analysis.

Through the assimilation of knowledge in system operation, computer operation, database management, and information management, the creation and operation of a successful program can be realized that addresses the tailored needs of society. A basic question centers on understanding how the computer works. The focus response is embedded in understanding the fetch-decode-execute cycle of the computer.

In this cycle, the computer first "fetches" the instruction (a series of binary codes) from memory. It then decodes the instruction, which means it interprets the binary code into something the computer can understand. Finally, the instruction is executed, which means that the computer actually carries out the instruction. This cycle is repeated continuously as long as the computer is powered on. Once the desired task is completed, desired information is stored, and the computer is turned off, the cycle ends for that task. The CPU is the brain of the operation. The computer is an intricate system composed of distinct parts and functions. The computer fetch-decode-execute cycle process is similar to the beginnings of the scientific problem-solving process, research process, algorithm process, and nursing process.

Critical Thought:
What Process Does This Cycle Remind You Of???

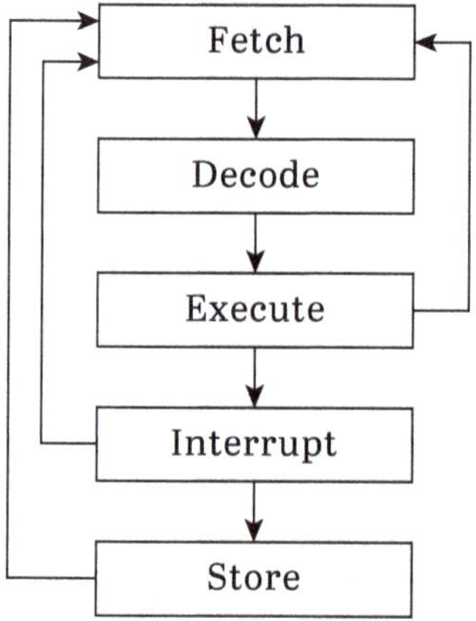

FIGURE 1.1 Fetch-decode-execute cycle

Health and HCIS

HCIS

A health information system (HIS) is a system that collects, manages, and uses health care data and information for decision-making, planning, and management of health care services. It can be defined as a set of interconnected components, including people, policies, procedures, and technologies, that work together to support the collection, processing, storage, retrieval, and analysis of health information for various purposes, such as clinical care, public health surveillance, research, and health system management. They can include EHRs, health information exchanges (HIEs), public health surveillance systems, disease registries, and other related systems.

A health care information system is a type of health information system that specifically focuses on the management and organization of health care information. The system captures, store, manages, and shares health care-related data and information to support the delivery of safe, effective, and efficient health care services. HIS include a variety of systems, such as EHRs, picture archiving and communication systems (PACS), laboratory information systems (LIS), pharmacy information systems (PIS), and other specialized systems used in health care settings. HIS plays a critical role in enabling health care providers to access and exchange patient information, make informed clinical decisions, and manage health care services more effectively.

Importance of HIS

HIS have the potential to provide many benefits to health care organizations and patients. One of the most significant benefits of HIS is improved quality of patient care. HIS can provide health care providers with immediate access to a patient's medical history, lab results, and other clinical information, enabling them to make better-informed decisions about patient care that leads to better patient outcomes.

HIS can also increase efficiency in health care organizations. By automating administrative tasks such as patient registration, scheduling, and billing, HIS can reduce the burden on health care staff and free up time to focus on patient care. HIS can also facilitate the sharing of information between different health care providers and organization networks, reducing duplication of effort and improving coordination of care. Another significant benefit of HIS is enhanced patient safety. HIS can help reduce errors in health care delivery by providing access to accurate and up-to-date patient information, supporting medication safety, and enabling real-time tracking of adverse events. This can help prevent harm to patients and improve overall patient safety.

Overall, the system serves as a tool that helps healthcare organizations monitor and improve the quality of care by providing access to data and analytics, tracking patient outcomes, ensuring safety, and enhancing satisfaction. HIS can improve financial performance by streamlining billing and reimbursement processes, reducing claim denials, and improving revenue cycle management. HIS can help health care organizations manage their finances more effectively, improving both the quality of care and financial management.

Examples of HIS Applications

These are just a few examples of the many HIS applications used in health care settings. Each HIS application has its own unique features and benefits, and together they form a complex ecosystem that supports the delivery of safe, effective, and efficient health care services.

HIS applications refer to various computer-based tools and technologies used in health care settings to improve patient care delivery, coordination, and outcomes. Some examples of HIS applications include EHRs and PACS.

Clinical decision support systems (CDSS) are computer programs that provide health care providers with information and recommendations to support clinical decision-making. CDSS can help prevent medication errors, diagnose medical conditions, and identify potential adverse events. HIEs are networks that enable the sharing of patient health information between different health care providers and organizations, improving care coordination, supporting public health surveillance, and facilitating research.

Telemedicine systems enable health care providers to deliver remote care to patients, using technologies such as videoconferencing, remote monitoring, and mobile health apps. Telemedicine systems can increase access to care, reduce health care costs, and improve patient outcomes.

Importance of Interoperability and Integration Between Different System Applications

Interoperability plays a critical role in HIS because it allows for seamless communication and sharing of data between different systems. For example, imagine a hospital that uses one system for their EHRs, another for their imaging systems, and yet another for their billing and financial systems. Without interoperability, these systems may not be able to communicate with each other, making it difficult to share important patient information or billing data. However, if these systems are interoperable, they can communicate and share data seamlessly, improving efficiency, reducing errors, and enabling better decision-making. This, in turn, can help health care providers deliver better patient care and improve the overall health care experience for patients.

Interoperability also plays a key role in health care data exchange between different health care organizations, such as hospitals, clinics, and other health care providers' networks. By enabling these organizations to exchange data seamlessly, interoperability can help improve patient outcomes and reduce health care costs by providing a more complete picture of a patient's health history.

Benefits of HIS

One key advantage of interoperability and integration is improved efficiency. When different systems can communicate with each other and share data seamlessly, it can reduce the need for manual data entry and other time-consuming tasks. This, in turn, can lead to improved productivity and efficiency. Another benefit of interoperability and integration is reduced errors. When data is manually entered into multiple systems, there is a higher risk of errors, such as typos or incorrect data. Interoperability and integration can help reduce these errors by automating data entry and ensuring that data is consistent across all systems.

Interoperability and integration can also enable better decision-making by providing a more complete picture of the data. For example, if financial data from an accounting system is integrated with sales data from a customer relationship management system, it can provide insights into how sales affect financial performance. This can help organizations make more informed decisions.

Improved customer experience is another benefit of interoperability and integration. By providing a seamless experience across different systems, organizations can improve the customer experience. For example, if a customer buys a product online, the order information can be seamlessly transferred to the shipping system to ensure timely delivery. Interoperability and integration provides flexibility and scalability by allowing different systems to be added or removed as needed. This can help organizations adapt to changing business needs and technological advancements.

Data Handling Management

Data handling management refers to the processes, procedures, and practices that are put in place to manage data effectively and efficiently throughout its lifecycle. It includes activities such as data collection, storage, analysis, dissemination, and disposal. The goal of data handling management is to ensure that data is accurate, reliable, secure, and accessible when needed. It involves developing and implementing policies and guidelines to govern data handling practices, as well as utilizing appropriate tools and technologies to support these practices. Effective data handling management is critical for organizations that rely on data to make informed decisions and achieve their objectives.

Structured Data

Structured data refers to data that is organized in a specific format that is easy to analyze and process. This type of data is typically stored in a relational database and is represented by tables with rows and columns. Structured data is characterized by a well-defined schema, or structure, that outlines the data elements, their attributes, and the relationships between them. Structured data can be easily queried, sorted, and analyzed using various tools and techniques, such as SQL queries, spreadsheets, or statistical software. Examples of structured data include financial transactions, customer information, or inventory records.

HOW TO DIFFERENTIATE KEY FEATURES OF STRUCTURED DATA

- It is organized and formatted in a consistent way.
- It can be easily queried, sorted, and analyzed using predefined rules and criteria.
- It is often machine readable, which means that it can be processed and analyzed automatically by software programs.
- It can be stored in a variety of formats, such as spreadsheets, databases, or XML files.

Unstructured Data

Unstructured data, on the other hand, refers to data that is not organized in a predefined or structured format. This type of data is often text heavy and lacks a consistent format or schema. Unstructured data can come from a variety of sources, such as social media posts, emails, customer feedback, or audio and video recordings. This data is often difficult to process and analyze using traditional tools and techniques, as it requires natural language processing (NLP) and machine learning (ML) algorithms to extract insights and meaning from it.

HOW TO DIFFERENTIATE KEY FEATURES OF UNSTRUCTURED DATA

- *Flexible schema*: Unlike structured databases that require a fixed schema to organize data, unstructured databases allow for a more flexible schema that can evolve over time. This enables organizations to add or modify data elements and attributes as needed, without disrupting the database structure.
- *Support for multiple data types*: Unstructured databases are designed to support a wide range of data types, including text, audio, images, and video. This enables organizations to store and analyze diverse data types in a single database.
- *Scalability*: Unstructured databases are designed to scale horizontally, which means that additional servers can be added to the database cluster to increase storage and processing capacity. This enables organizations to handle large volumes of data and accommodate future growth.
- *Searchability*: Unstructured databases often provide advanced search capabilities that allow users to search for specific data elements or patterns within the data. This is particularly useful for organizations that need to analyze large volumes of text data, such as customer feedback or social media posts.

- *Integration with NLP and ML tools*: Unstructured databases often provide integration with NLP and ML tools, which enable organizations to analyze and extract insights from unstructured data. This can include sentiment analysis, topic modeling, and image recognition.
- *Cloud-based deployment*: Many unstructured databases are designed to be deployed in the cloud, which provides flexibility and scalability. Cloud-based deployment also enables organizations to access and analyze data from anywhere with an internet connection.

In summary, unstructured databases are designed to support diverse data types and enable flexible schema and scalability. They often provide advanced search capabilities and integration with NLP and ML tools and are frequently deployed in the cloud.

Importance of Data Management in Health Care

Database management plays a crucial role in health care by efficiently managing patient data, which includes medical histories, test results, treatment plans, and other critical information. An efficient database management system (DBMS) ensures that this data is organized, stored securely, and easily accessible when needed. By having a comprehensive DBMS in place, health care providers can access critical information about their patients quickly and efficiently. This can lead to faster and more accurate diagnoses, improved treatment plans, and ultimately better patient outcomes.

Moreover, health care organizations are subject to numerous regulatory requirements that dictate how patient data must be collected, stored, and shared. A robust DBMS can help ensure compliance with these requirements, protecting patient privacy and avoiding legal and financial penalties. When properly managed, health data is a valuable resource for research and analysis. A well-designed DBMS can support research efforts by providing a centralized repository of data that can be analyzed and mined for insights. In conclusion, database management is critical for health care organizations to efficiently manage patient data, improve patient outcomes, ensure regulatory compliance, and support research and analysis efforts.

Tools and Techniques for Managing Data

There are several tools and techniques available for managing data in health care and other industries. The most common type of database used is a relational database, which stores data in tables with predefined relationships between them. This makes it easy to search, sort, and manipulate data. Another tool used for managing data is a data warehouse, which is a large-scale repository that collects and stores data from multiple sources. Data warehouses support analytics and reporting and are optimized for querying and analysis.

Data integration tools are also used to integrate data from different sources, formats, and platforms. They can transform data into a common format and map data elements between systems. Another important tool for managing data is data modeling, which is the process of creating a conceptual representation of data objects, relationships between them, and rules for their use. Data modeling helps to ensure that data is structured in a way that supports business requirements and is consistent across the organization. Data quality management is critical for ensuring that data is accurate, complete, and consistent. Data quality management tools help to identify and correct errors and inconsistencies in data. Data security tools are also important for protecting data from unauthorized access, use, or disclosure. These tools include access controls, encryption, firewalls, and other security measures.

Finally, data governance is the process of defining and implementing policies and procedures for managing data across the organization. It involves establishing standards for data quality, security, privacy, and compliance and ensuring that they are followed. The tools and techniques for managing data in health care and other industries include relational databases, data warehouses, data integration tools, data modeling, data quality management, data security tools, and data governance. Each of these tools plays a critical role in ensuring that data is managed effectively and efficiently.

Information System Configuration

Information system configuration refers to the process of setting up and arranging the different components that make up an information system. An information system typically includes hardware components such as servers, storage devices, and network devices, as well as software components such as operating systems, databases, and application software. Configuring an information system involves selecting the appropriate hardware and software components, connecting them, and setting them up to work together seamlessly. In addition to selecting and configuring the components, information system configuration also involves setting up security measures to protect the system from cyberattacks and data breaches. This can include setting up firewalls, antivirus software, access controls, and other security measures.

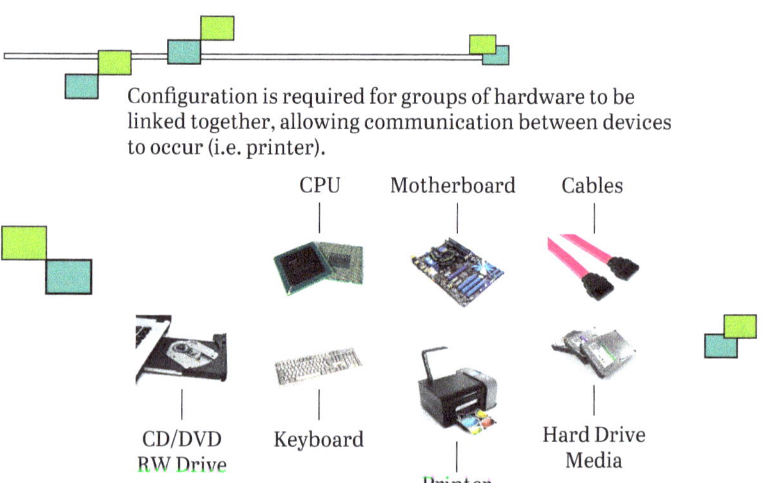

FIGURE 1.2 Systems configuration.

Scalability is another important aspect of information system configuration. Organizations need information systems that can grow and adapt to changing business needs over time. A well-configured information system should be able to accommodate growth and expansion and should be designed with future needs in mind.

Finally, information system configuration also involves planning for ongoing maintenance and support. A properly configured information system requires regular maintenance to ensure that it continues to operate smoothly and efficiently. It should also be designed with supportability in mind so that any issues that arise can be quickly and easily addressed.

Overall, information system configuration is a critical process that requires careful planning and attention to detail. A well-configured information system can help organizations operate more efficiently and effectively, while also reducing the risk of security breaches and other disruptions.

Importance of Configuration in Health Care

Configuration is a critical aspect of HCIS, given the complexity and sensitivity of health care systems. HCIS must be able to handle large amounts of data while also ensuring patient data is kept confidential and secure. Therefore, proper configuration of health care systems is necessary to ensure that the systems operate efficiently, effectively, and securely. One of the key benefits of configuration in health care is improved patient care. Proper configuration of health care systems helps health care providers access and analyze patient data quickly and accurately, leading to better diagnoses and treatment decisions. Configuration can also improve communication among health care providers, leading to better coordination of care and improved patient outcomes.

Configuration also helps health care providers spend more time focusing on patient care by streamlining workflows and automating routine tasks. This reduces costs, increases productivity, and improves overall operational efficiency. Moreover, proper configuration of health care systems is essential for ensuring the security and privacy of patient data. Health care systems that are not properly configured can be vulnerable to cyberattacks and data breaches, compromising patient confidentiality and leading to legal and financial consequences. Therefore, proper configuration of health care systems includes setting up security protocols such as firewalls, access controls, and encryption to protect patient data from unauthorized access.

Proper configuration of health care systems is essential for ensuring high-quality patient care, improving efficiency, and protecting patient data. Health care organizations that invest in configuration can expect to see benefits in the form of improved patient outcomes, increased productivity, enhanced security, and financial return on investment. It is therefore critical for health care informatics graduate-level students to learn about the importance of configuration in HCIS:

- *Conduct a thorough needs assessment*: Before configuring a HCIS, it is important to conduct a thorough needs assessment to understand the organization's requirements, workflows, and data management needs.
- *Plan for scalability*: Health care organizations should plan for future growth and expansion when configuring information systems to ensure that the systems can accommodate increasing volumes of data and users.
- *Standardize processes*: Standardizing processes can help ensure consistency and reduce errors in data entry and management. Health care organizations should strive to standardize data elements, workflows, and processes across all departments and systems.
- *Ensure data quality*: Health care organizations should establish processes for ensuring the quality of data entered into information systems, such as data validation and error checking.
- *Implement security measures*: Health care organizations must take steps to ensure the security and privacy of patient data. This includes implementing security protocols such as firewalls, access controls, and encryption.

- *Train users*: Health care organizations should provide comprehensive training to users of information systems to ensure that they can use the systems effectively and efficiently.
- *Regularly review and update configurations*: HCIS should be regularly reviewed and updated to ensure that they continue to meet the organization's needs and comply with regulatory requirements.

By following these best practices, health care organizations can configure information systems that support high-quality patient care, improve efficiency, and protect patient data.

Summary

In summation, this chapter provided an overview of HIS and their importance in health care. It explained the basic components of a computer system, introduced different HIS applications, and covered data handling/management, including the types of data, the importance of data management, and the tools and techniques for managing data. It presented different health care systems and emphasized the importance of interoperability and integration. The chapter concluded with explaining the concept of information system configuration and its importance in health care, identifying the components of an information system configuration, and providing best practices for configuring HCIS. Overall, the chapter highlighted the critical role of HIS and its components, functions, and management in supporting efficient and effective health care delivery.

The constructivism of learning HCIS, computer systems, interoperability, integration, database management, structured data, unstructured data, configuration, information management, health-related programs, data sources, data elements, database schemas, and data analysis will lead to the end goals related to the creation of mobile technology, enhancement of access to quality health care, heightened sustainability, patients' being self-managers of care, and advanced fiscal and project management in the varied health venues.

Chapter Review Questions

Directions: Consider what you learned in this chapter as you respond to the health care scenario and questions.

Health Care Scenario: Navigating Health Care System Upgrades

Dr. Jones is a health care informatics specialist working in a large hospital. The hospital has recently decided to upgrade its HIS to improve patient care and streamline operations. Dr. Jones's role is to ensure that the new system integrates seamlessly with the hospital's existing data and enhances its functionality.

As part of the upgrade process, Dr. Jones encounters several challenges and questions. Let's see how well you can help Dr. Jones by answering these questions correctly!

Multiple-Choice Questions

1. Dr. Jones wants to ensure that the new HIS will integrate various health care processes efficiently. What is the main advantage of an HIS?
   a. It simplifies patient care.
   b. It reduces health care costs.
   c. It ensures data security.
   d. It integrates various health care processes efficiently.
2. While setting up the new system, Dr. Jones needs to understand which component is responsible for executing software instructions. Which component of a computer system is responsible for this?
   a. Hardware
   b. Data
   c. Software
   d. Operating system

3. Dr. Jones is explaining to the hospital staff the benefits of the new HIS. What is a primary benefit of an HIS?

    a. It reduces the need for health care professionals.
    b. It improves patient outcomes through better data management.
    c. It eliminates all errors in medical records.
    d. It is cheaper than traditional health care methods.

4. During training, Dr. Jones emphasizes the importance of data management. What distinguishes structured data from unstructured data?

    a. Structured data is unorganized and hard to analyze.
    b. Structured data can be easily queried and sorted.
    c. Unstructured data is always machine readable.
    d. Unstructured data is stored in spreadsheets and databases.

5. To manage the hospital's vast amount of data, Dr. Jones recommends using a specific tool. Which tool is commonly used for managing health care data?

    a. Word processors
    b. Database management systems
    c. Email servers
    d. Web browsers

6. Dr. Jones explains to the IT team why interoperability is crucial for the new HIS. Why is interoperability important in health care systems?

    a. It allows for the replacement of health care professionals.
    b. It ensures that data is encrypted.
    c. It facilitates seamless communication and data exchange between systems.
    d. It reduces the amount of data stored.

By understanding and applying these principles, Dr. Jones successfully upgrades the hospital's HIS, leading to improved efficiency, better patient outcomes, and a more integrated health care delivery system.

Answer Key

1. (d) It integrates various health care processes efficiently.
2. (a) Hardware
3. (b) It improves patient outcomes through better data management.
4. (b) Structured data can be easily queried and sorted.
5. (b) Database management systems
6. (c) It facilitates seamless communication and data exchange between systems.

References

Dee, C. R. (2007). The development of the Medical Literature Analysis and Retrieval System (MEDLARS). *Journal of the Library Association, 95*(4), 416–25.

Gagne, R. M. (1985). The events of instruction. In R. M. Gagne (Ed.), *The conditions of learning and theory of instruction* (4th ed., pp. 29–56). Holt, Rinehart & Winston.

Reznick, J. (2017, August 2). *A new history of NLM: Celebrating 150 years of public service and looking to the future*. National Library of Medicine. https://circulatingnow.nlm.nih.gov/2017/08/02/new-history-of-the-nlm-celebrating-150-years-of-public-service-and-looking-to-the-future/

Figure Credits

Chapter 2

Advancing Patient Care Through Technology and Algorithmic Solutions

Introduction

The purpose of Chapter 2 is to examine how technological innovations are transforming health care. Specifically, this chapter will explore the impact of algorithms in creating personalized interventions, optimizing treatment plans, and enhancing diagnostic accuracy. These algorithms play a crucial role in personalizing health care experiences, significantly improving patient outcomes.

Additionally, Chapter 2 will introduce the advancements in robotics and remote monitoring technologies. These innovations provide more precise and timely care, particularly benefiting individuals in remote or underserved areas.

By delving into the intricate landscape of health care technology, this chapter will highlight the potential of these advancements to revolutionize patient care, improve accessibility, and optimize health care systems. Moving beyond foundational concepts, the focus will be on the dynamic and transformative aspects of technology that empower and engage patients.

The significance of Chapter 2 lies in its focus on the crucial role of patient engagement in modern health care. It underscores the shift from a one-sided approach to a collaborative effort between patients and providers. By empowering patients to take an active role in their care through personalized health management systems and biometric authentication, the chapter illustrates how these technologies make managing health easier and more secure, leading to better health outcomes and a more satisfying health care experience.

Importantly, the chapter also addresses the complexities and ethical considerations of these technological advancements. It thoughtfully discusses concerns about patient privacy and the potential risks of algorithmic applications, ensuring the conversation remains grounded in real-world implications. The chapter emphasizes that the well-being and privacy of patients must be prioritized, reinforcing that technological progress should uphold ethical standards.

In essence, Chapter 2 offers an insightful look at the future of health care, whereby technology and human interaction come together to create a more effective and compassionate system. By exploring these innovative approaches, the chapter aims to give readers a deeper understanding of how technology can transform health care, ultimately leading to better health outcomes and a more inclusive, efficient health care system.

Objectives That Lead to Outcomes

We have detailed specific goals and the expected outcomes. The following table aligns these key objectives with their corresponding outcomes, offering a clear and comprehensive understanding of what learners should achieve and comprehend upon completion. This alignment ensures that each objective is paired with a tangible and measurable outcome, thereby enhancing the overall learning experience. By presenting the objectives alongside their connected outcomes in a clear and structured manner, the table highlights the intended impacts of each initiative.

Objective	Outcome
Develop and apply algorithms to improve medical diagnoses and treatments, identify patterns and trends, and enhance patient care and outcomes in telemedicine and remote consultations.	Improved accuracy in medical diagnoses and treatments, better identification of patterns and trends in patient data, enhanced patient care and outcomes in telemedicine and remote consultations.

Empower patients to manage their health through self-manager devices and resources.	Promoted self-care, reduced health care costs, and increased patient engagement in their own health management.
Enhance surgical precision and provide rehabilitation and assistance with daily living activities through robotics.	Reduced health care costs through automation of certain tasks and procedures, improved surgical outcomes, and better support for rehabilitation and daily living activities.
Improve access to health care services and monitor chronic conditions in real time through remote monitoring technology.	Reduced need for in-person consultations and hospitalizations, better management of chronic conditions, and increased accessibility to health care services.
Promote healthy aging and prevent or delay the onset of chronic conditions through lifestyle changes and personalized health management plans and resources.	Improved health outcomes for the aging population, delayed onset of chronic conditions, and increased adoption of healthier lifestyles.
Enhance patient security and privacy through biometric authentication.	Improved security and privacy for patient data, better monitoring of health indicators, and comprehensive analysis of population health trends and patterns.
Improve communication and collaboration between health care providers through secure networks and information exchange systems.	Enhanced access and sharing of patient data and medical records, improved health care efficiency, and reduced administrative costs through automation of certain tasks.

Key Terms

Directions: Before reading, please look at this list of key terms that will be used in this chapter. If any term is unfamiliar, please see the glossary at the end of the book.

algorithms
biometrics
improve outcomes
networks
remote monitoring
robotics
self-managers

Enhancing Medical Diagnostics and Treatments

Importance of Technology in Health Care

The advancement in health care has a long-standing history, continuously building phenomenal technology to improve outcomes. Throughout history, remarkable inventors and organizations have made significant contributions. Hippocrates, the "father of medicine," established medical ethics and a systematic approach. Ibn al-Nafis challenged prevailing ideas with his description of pulmonary circulation (West, 2008). René Laennec revolutionized diagnosis with the stethoscope (Roguin, 2006). Wilhelm Roentgen's discovery of X-rays enabled noninvasive imaging. Alexander Fleming's discovery of penicillin transformed bacterial infection treatment. In recent times, inventors like Robert S. Ledley and Sir Godfrey Hounsfield developed computed tomography (CT) scanning technology, providing detailed cross-sectional imaging (Sittig et al., 2006). Raymond Damadian invented the magnetic resonance imaging (MRI) scanner for noninvasive visualization. Notable organizations like Apple and Medtronic have also made significant contributions. Apple's Apple Watch incorporates heart rate monitoring, electrocardiogram (ECG) capabilities, and fall detection (Perez et al., 2019). Medtronic has advanced various areas with devices for cardiac and neurostimulation, insulin pumps, and surgical robotics. These inventors, organizations, and their contributions represent a fraction of the remarkable individuals and teams working to improve health care technology.

Advanced technology has ushered in a new era in health care, revolutionizing the industry and bringing numerous advantages that significantly improve patient care and outcomes. Enhanced diagnostics is a key benefit. Imaging techniques like MRI, CT, and positron emission tomography (PET) provide detailed images, aiding in detection and diagnosis. Sophisticated laboratory tests and genetic screenings enable earlier disease identification and personalized treatment plans.

The latest technologies in health care include telemedicine, wearable devices, AI, robotics, 3D printing, EHRs, precision medicine, and augmented reality and virtual reality (AR/VR). Telemedicine allows remote doctor consultations, wearable devices track vital signs and manage chronic conditions, AI analyzes patient data for personalized treatment, robotics assist with surgery and rehabilitation, 3D printing creates customized medical devices, EHRs provide easy access to patient information, precision medicine tailors treatments to genetic makeup, and AR/VR are used for medical training and patient education. These technologies have evolved over decades, with telemedicine and EHRs becoming more widespread due to the COVID-19 pandemic. New advances will continue to transform health care in years to come.

The advancements in technology have empowered patients to take an active role in managing their health. Smartphone apps, wearable devices, and online platforms provide individuals with tools to monitor their fitness, nutrition, and overall well-being. These technologies offer personalized recommendations, track progress, and promote healthy lifestyle behaviors. Access to online health information and tele-education platforms enables patients to educate themselves about medical conditions, preventive measures, and treatment options, empowering them to make informed decisions about their care.

Overall, advanced technology has brought about significant benefits to the health care industry, thanks in part to the crucial role played by informaticists. Advancements in medicine, guided by informaticists, have transformed patient care through enhanced diagnostics, precision medicine, minimally invasive procedures, telemedicine, and patient empowerment. These advancements have led to improved outcomes and contributed to the overall advancement and patient satisfaction. Developing mastery of the technology is instrumental in optimizing the use of technology and facilitating the exchange of health information, ultimately enabling health care professionals to make informed decisions, improving patient outcomes, and advancing the field of medicine to new heights.

TABLE 2.1 The Major Benefit of the Listed Latest Technology Used in Health Care

Latest Technology	Virtual Visit	Tailored Treatmentt	Virtual Treatment Training and Education	Remote Consult	Monitor Vital Signs	Analyze Patient Data	Develop Treatment Plan	Assist With Surgery and Rehab	Create Medical Device	Provide Easy Access to Patient Information
Telemedicine	★			★						
Wearable Devices					★					
Artificial Intelligence (AI)						★	★			
Robotics								★		
3D Printing									★	
Electronic Health Record										★
Precision Medicine		★								
Augmented Reality			★							
Virtual Reality			★							

Algorithm Development and Application

An algorithm is a step-by-step procedure or set of rules designed to solve a specific problem or accomplish a particular task. It is a precise, well-defined sequence of instructions that takes an input, processes it, and produces an output. Algorithms can be expressed in various forms, such as natural language, pseudocode, flowcharts, or programming languages.

The goal of an algorithm is to provide a clear and unambiguous solution to a problem, ensuring that if followed correctly, it will produce the desired result for any valid input. Algorithms are fundamental to computer science and are used in various fields, including mathematics, engineering, data analysis, AI, and more.

Key characteristics of algorithms include their correctness, efficiency, and generality. Correctness refers to the algorithm's ability to produce the correct output for any valid input. Efficiency relates to the algorithm's ability to solve the problem with optimal use of resources, such as time (the amount of computational time or the number of operations an algorithm needs to complete its task) and memory (the amount of computer memory or storage space an algorithm needs to store and manipulate data during its execution). Generality means that an algorithm should be applicable to a wide range of input instances rather than specific to a particular case.

Improve Medical Diagnostic and Treatment

Overall, algorithms are essential tools for solving problems and serve as the building blocks for developing software, creating efficient processes, and advancing computational capabilities. Conceptually, algorithms follow the same process related to the scientific problem-solving process, research process, and nursing process, starting with the identification of a problem.

As informaticists, our goal is to leverage algorithms to develop a comprehensive plan for addressing health problems within a given population. To achieve this, we start by collecting data on societal health issues, with a particular focus on the demographics of the target population. We gather information such as the nature of the problem;

attributes related to the problem; and demographics related to the target population, such as names, health problems, educational levels, ages, and other relevant factors. Understanding the demographics of the population provides valuable insights into the key variables that contribute to the overall health challenges they face. By employing algorithms and data-mining techniques, we can analyze the captured data to build descriptive and predictive models. Informaticists are instrumental in the collection and analysis of demographic and health-related data. They play a vital role in identifying crucial variables and patterns through data-mining techniques, informing the decision-making process. These experts utilize algorithms as instructions for processing the data, enabling them to build descriptive and predictive models that guide the development of effective solutions to the health problems faced by the target population.

Informaticists bring their specialized knowledge and skills to the table, driving the data-driven plan for addressing health problems. Their expertise in algorithms and data mining empowers them to extract valuable insights and patterns from complex datasets, leading to informed decision-making and the development of tailored solutions. By collaborating with health care professionals, informaticists play a pivotal role in improving the health outcomes of the target population.

THE STEPS TO FOLLOW WHEN CREATING AN ALGORITHM, ALONG WITH THE CORRESPONDING FLOWCHART SYMBOLS

Understand the Problem

- Define the problem you want to solve and clearly understand its requirements.
- Identify the main tasks or sub-problems that need to be addressed.
- Define inputs and outputs.
- Determine what data or information is needed as input and what should be produced as output.
- Plan the solution steps.

- Outline the high-level steps required to solve the problem.
- Determine the outcome.

Commonly Used Flowchart Symbols

- Terminal/start/end: Represents the beginning or end of the program. **Symbol: Oval**
- Input/output: Represents the input or output of data. **Symbol: Parallelogram**
- Process/operation: Represents a specific action or operation to be performed. **Symbol: Rectangle**
- Decision: Represents a conditional statement or decision point. **Symbol: Diamond**
- Connector/off-page connector: Connects different sections of the flowchart or indicates a continuation on another page. **Symbol: Circle**

Connect the Symbols

- Connect the flowchart symbols using **arrows** to indicate the flow of control or data between different steps.
- Validate and refine.
- Review the flowchart and algorithm to ensure correctness and efficiency.
- Make any necessary improvements or adjustments
- Implement the algorithm.

It's important to note that flowchart symbols may vary slightly depending on the conventions used, but the ones mentioned are commonly used and should provide a good starting point. Remember, the specific steps and symbols used will depend on the complexity and nature of the problem you are trying to solve.

Algorithm Application

Problem: Impending hospital closure servicing the communities of Central Brooklyn. The hospital averages 70,000 annual visits for chronic disease of the elderly, diabetes, hypertension, and obesity. The population consists of uninsured and underinsured clients.

Objective: Consider alternative means to address the health care needs of the community. How would you use an algorithm to solve the problem of inaccessible health care monitoring services for a population with congestive heart failure (CHF), diabetes mellitus (DM), and chronic obstructive pulmonary disease (COPD) due to the closing of their community-based hospital?

Table 2.1 reflects some of the common symbols used in flowcharts to create an algorithm. However, it's worth noting that the specific symbols used can vary depending on the conventions followed by different organizations or individuals.

TABLE 2.1 Applying an Algorithm: A Step-by-Step Approach

Name	Symbol	Purpose	Process Illustration
Start/End		The oval represents a start and end point: Start with the problem.	Community hospital closes
Parallelo-gram		The parallelogram represents the input or output of data.	Population of elderly residents with chronic health problems (CHF, DM, COPD) need monitoring
Decision Point / Decision Symbol		The diamond represents a decision point when the algorithm evaluates a condition and selects different paths based on the result. Typically, there are two arrows coming out of the decision symbol, one for yes and another for no, leading to different parts of the flowchart.	Available resources, modes of delivery

Process/ Action	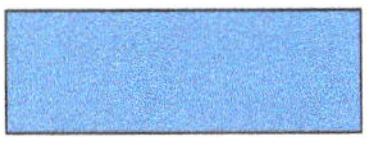	The rectangle represents a specific action or process that occurs in the algorithm. It can include calculations, operations, or any other action that transforms or manipulates data.	Contact for viable resources using technology
Double Sided-Rectangle Predefined Process	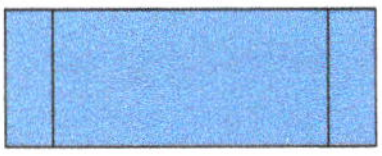	The double-sided rectangle represents a process or action that is predefined and already defined elsewhere in the algorithm. Modules or subordinates expressed elsewhere.	CHF: Monday, DM: Wednesday, COPD: Thursday; predefined process steps
Hexagon for Loop		The hexagon shows the initiation of a loop.	Replicates the predefined process weekly; looping
Circle	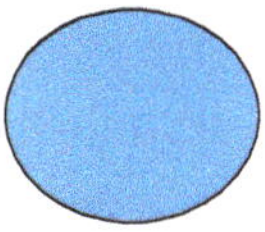	The circle represents the connector symbol, which is used to connect different parts of the flowchart when the algorithm continues on another page or is split across multiple sections.	Connector for patient health care provider and technology
Flow		Joins two symbols and shows the flow	Continued flow direction

Self-Managers of Care

Self-managers of care refer to individuals who take an active role in managing their own health care and well-being. These individuals assume responsibility for making informed decisions about their health, coordinating their care, and implementing strategies to maintain or improve their overall well-being.

In a health care setting, patients are no longer passive recipients of care but active participants in their own well-being. They become self-managers of care by utilizing devices, applications, or programs that assist them in managing their health and wellness. These tools offer various functionalities such as tracking and monitoring health indicators, scheduling appointments, setting goals, and accessing resources and support.

To enhance self-management abilities, patients are provided with opportunities for skill-building and support. Education sessions, workshops, and one-on-one coaching are offered to develop problem-solving techniques, effective communication skills, and decision-making strategies. Patients also benefit from support networks, such as peer support groups or online communities, giving them spaces where they can share experiences, exchange knowledge, and provide mutual encouragement.

Continuous follow-up and evaluation are vital for ongoing support. Health care providers regularly check in with patients to assess their progress, address concerns, and provide guidance. Patients are encouraged to keep track of their health indicators, symptoms, or medication adherence. This self-awareness enables informed discussions with health care providers and fosters a sense of empowerment.

In today's health care landscape, technology plays a significant role in empowering individuals to self-manage their care effectively and adds a new dimension to the self-management journey. Through the integration of digital tools, an empowering mindset is further fostered, aligning seamlessly with the principles mentioned above.

Health informatics specialists work to develop and implement various devices, applications, and programs that assist individuals in self-managing their care. They collaborate with health care providers to design tools for tracking and monitoring health indicators, scheduling appointments, setting goals, and accessing resources and support. These experts ensure that these technological solutions align with the specific needs and goals of patients, making it easier for them to take control of their health and well-being.

Mobile apps and digital platforms enable seamless communication and collaboration between health care providers and patients. Secure messaging systems allow patients to ask questions, report symptoms, or request prescription refills conveniently. Telemedicine and virtual visits provide opportunities for remote consultations, eliminating the need for in-person appointments and making health care more accessible, especially for those with mobility or transportation limitations.

Technology also enables personalized reminders and notifications to help patients stay on track with their self-management routines. Medication reminder apps can alert patients to take their medications at the prescribed times. Activity trackers can provide reminders to engage in physical activity or take breaks during sedentary periods. These prompts support patients in adhering to their self-care regimens and maintaining consistency.

Furthermore, technology facilitates peer support and community engagement. Online forums, social media groups, and virtual support communities connect patients with others who share similar health concerns. These platforms provide opportunities for sharing experiences, seeking advice, and offering mutual support. Patients can learn from one another, gain insights into different self-management strategies, and find a sense of belonging within a community of like-minded individuals.

Data analytics and AI have the potential to revolutionize self-management by providing personalized insights and recommendations. By analyzing large datasets, AI algorithms can identify patterns, predict outcomes, and offer tailored recommendations for self-care. This includes proactive suggestions, reminders, and educational materials based on patients' specific needs, preferences, and health history.

Integrating technology in self-management requires ensuring privacy, security, and digital literacy. Health care providers and technology developers must prioritize data protection, secure communication channels, and user-friendly interfaces. Patient education on digital literacy and responsible technology use is essential to empower individuals to effectively navigate and leverage these tools.

Embracing the meaningful use of technology enables patients to access information, connect with health care providers, track progress, and engage in self-management in unprecedented ways. Technology expands the possibilities for personalized care, promotes patient autonomy, and ultimately improves health outcomes.

Health informatics specialists develop and implement various devices, applications, and programs that assist individuals in self-managing their care.

Advantages of Self-Management of Care

As health care continues to evolve, self-management has emerged as a valuable approach that empowers individuals to take an active role in their well-being. By engaging in self-care practices and making informed decisions about their health, patients can experience a range of benefits that enhance their overall quality of life. The following are key advantages of self-management of care:

- *Increased autonomy*: Self-managers of care have greater control over their health care decisions and treatment plans. They can actively participate in their care and have a say in determining the best course of action for their well-being.
- *Enhanced patient–provider collaboration*: Self-management encourages a collaborative relationship between patients and health care providers. It fosters open communication, trust, and shared decision-making, leading to better health care outcomes.
- *Improved health outcomes*: Patients who take an active role in managing their care tend to experience better health outcomes. They are more likely to adhere to treatment plans, engage in preventive measures, and make healthier lifestyle choices.

- *Better understanding of personal health*: Self-managers of care develop a deeper understanding of their health conditions, symptoms, and treatment options. This knowledge empowers them to make informed decisions and take proactive steps to maintain their well-being.
- *Cost-effectiveness*: Self-management of care can potentially reduce health care costs. By actively managing their health, patients may avoid unnecessary hospital visits, emergency room trips, and complications, leading to overall cost savings.

Disadvantages of Self-Management of Care

While self-management of care offers many benefits, it also comes with certain challenges that can impact a patient's ability to manage their health effectively. Without the necessary knowledge, resources, and support, self-managing care can become overwhelming and, in some cases, lead to unintended consequences. The following are key disadvantages of self-management of care:

- *Lack of expertise*: Patients may not possess the necessary medical knowledge and expertise to fully manage their care. They might face challenges in interpreting complex medical information, making accurate decisions, or identifying potential risks or complications.
- *Limited access to resources*: Self-management relies on access to resources such as reliable health care information, support networks, and digital tools. Not all individuals may have equal access to these resources, leading to disparities in self-management capabilities.
- *Emotional burden*: Taking on the responsibility of self-management can be emotionally challenging for some individuals. Coping with chronic conditions, adhering to treatment plans, and making health care decisions can cause stress, anxiety, and feelings of being overwhelmed.
- *Risk of misinformation*: With the abundance of health information available online, patients may encounter conflicting or inaccurate information. This can lead to confusion, misguided decisions, or the adoption of potentially harmful practices.

- *Time and effort requirements*: Effective self-management requires time and effort on the part of the patient. It involves learning about the condition, monitoring symptoms, adhering to treatment plans, and incorporating lifestyle changes. This can be demanding and may affect the patient's daily routines and quality of life.

It is crucial to emphasize that self-management of care should be complemented by a collaborative relationship with health care providers. While patients can take an active role in managing their care, health care professionals play a vital role in providing guidance, expertise, and monitoring to ensure optimal outcomes. Together, patients and health care providers can work hand in hand to achieve the best possible health outcomes and enhance the overall well-being of individuals.

Robotics and Health Care

Robotics is the use of mechanical or electronic devices capable of performing complex or repetitive tasks automatically, either independently or under human control. In health care, robotics can be used for a variety of purposes, such as surgery, rehabilitation, and assistance with daily living activities.

Robotics

In the vast realm of health care, a technological revolution has been unfolding, a revolution powered by the relentless march of robotics. Picture a world in which machines work alongside skilled medical professionals, augmenting their abilities and transforming the landscape of patient care.

The seeds of this revolution were sown many decades ago when pioneers began to explore the potential of merging technology and medicine. The earliest inklings of robotic systems in health care emerged in the 1980s, when researchers laid the foundation for what would become a remarkable journey of innovation.

Robotic surgery burst onto the scene, captivating the imaginations of medical professionals and patients alike. Surgeons embraced the prospect of tiny robotic assistants, their nimble "hands" guided by the deft touch of a human operator. These robotics surgical systems granted surgeons a newfound precision, enabling intricate procedures with minimal invasiveness, reduced scarring, and swifter recoveries.

As the technology advanced, so did its capabilities. The robotic revolution extended its reach into the realm of rehabilitation. Patients grappling with physical impairments found hope in the form of robotic companions. These machines tirelessly worked with individuals, helping them regain their motor functions, strengthen weakened muscles, and reclaim their independence.

Telepresence robots emerged, a beacon of connectivity in an ever-expanding world. These robotic marvels facilitated virtual consultations, bridging the distances that once separated patients from health care providers. With their cameras, microphones, and screens, telepresence robots brought the healing touch of doctors to remote corners of the globe, providing expert care and guidance to those who needed it most.

Robotic prosthetics, another triumph of this revolution, unlocked a world of possibilities for amputees. These mechanical limbs, imbued with intelligence and grace, seamlessly integrated with the human body. Sensors and algorithms worked in harmony, translating nerve impulses into fluid movements, giving amputees a second chance at life. With robotic prosthetics, they could once again grasp a loved one's hand, climb mountains, and dance under the stars. Automation became the new norm, as robots deftly handled medication dispensing, laboratory testing, and inventory management. Accuracy soared, errors diminished, and health care professionals had more time to devote to patient care.

The journey didn't end there. Robotic exoskeletons arrived, standing as beacons of strength and resilience. These wearable wonders provided support to patients with mobility impairments, giving them the power to walk tall once more. Health care workers, burdened by heavy lifting tasks, found solace in the mechanical arms of exoskeletons, sharing the load and preserving their own well-being.

Robotics in health care are continuing to unfold, weaving together technological marvels with the art of healing. From the early days of robotic surgery to the present era of telepresence, prosthetics, and automation, robots had become trusted companions to health care professionals, forever altering the landscape of patient care.

As the future unfolds, the journey of robotics in health care continues. Boundaries will be shattered, new horizons will be explored, and the world of medicine will be forever transformed by the embrace of technology. In this extraordinary fusion of robotics and health care, hope thrives, lives are changed, and the promise of a healthier, brighter future awaits.

Advantages of Robotics in Health Care

In the bustling world of health care, where every second counts and lives hang in the balance, robotics emerged as a formidable ally, armed with an array of advantages that revolutionized the way medicine was practiced:

- In the realm of rehabilitation, the advantages of robotics were equally profound. Imagine a determined patient, their body weakened by injury or disability, guided by a robotic companion. With tireless persistence, these machines facilitated repetitive movements, guiding patients along the path of recovery. The advantages were clear: improved motor function, strengthened muscles, and restored independence. Patients regained hope, and their spirits lifted as they witnessed the transformative power of these robotic allies.
- Telepresence robots brought forth a new era of connectivity and accessibility. The advantages were palpable as doctors, armed with cameras and screens, transcended geographical barriers to reach patients in far-flung corners of the world. Remote consultations became a reality, enabling timely diagnosis, expert guidance, and personalized care. For patients who were once isolated or lacked access to specialized health care,

the advantages were immeasurable—the healing touch of a physician was just a video call away.

- The advantages of robotic prosthetics were nothing short of life changing. Picture an amputee, who once grappled with the loss of a limb, stepping into a new world of possibilities. With robotic limbs, the advantages were clear—enhanced functionality, natural movements, and restored mobility. These mechanical marvels breathed life into their wearers, empowering them to grasp, walk, and dance once more. The advantages were not merely physical; they extended to the realm of emotional well-being, fostering a sense of wholeness and renewed confidence.
- Automation in pharmacies and laboratories brought about a plethora of advantages. Robots expertly handled medication dispensing, eliminating errors and improving accuracy. In laboratories, the advantages were twofold; robots performed repetitive tasks with unwavering precision, while freeing up health care professionals to focus on complex analyses and patient care. Efficiency soared, errors dwindled, and the advantages were evident in the seamless flow of health care delivery.
- Imagine a bustling operating room, where a surgeon's hands deftly maneuver robotic instruments with precision and grace. The advantages of robotic surgery became apparent as incisions shrank, blood loss diminished, and recovery times accelerated. Surgeons reveled in the enhanced visualization and dexterity afforded by these mechanical marvels, while patients rejoiced at the prospect of faster healing, reduced pain, and minimized scarring.

Disadvantages of Robotics in Health Care

As with any revolutionary advancement, the world of robotics in health care also bore its share of disadvantages, casting a shadow amidst the dazzling array of advantages:

- In the realm of robotic surgery, the disadvantages often center around the high costs involved. The sophisticated technology requires hefty investments, making it inaccessible for many health care institutions. Additionally, the steep learning curve for surgeons poses challenges, as acquiring the necessary skills and expertise takes time and resources. Moreover, the reliance on technology introduces an element of vulnerability: Technical malfunctions or errors in programming could potentially compromise patient safety.

- Robotic rehabilitation, though promising, has its drawbacks. The cost of these machines limits their widespread adoption, making them accessible to only a fortunate few. While the repetitive movements facilitated by robots are beneficial, some critics argue that the human touch and personalized care of health care professionals can never be fully replaced. The question of whether robots can truly replicate the empathy and emotional support required for rehabilitation remains an ongoing debate.
- Telepresence robots, while expanding the reach of health care, present their own set of disadvantages. Connectivity issues and technological limitations occasionally hinder the quality of virtual consultations, leaving room for misinterpretation or incomplete assessments. Furthermore, the absence of physical presence during examinations means that certain aspects of patient evaluation, such as palpation or hands-on assessments, are compromised. The advantages of remote care are not without their trade-offs.
- Robotic prosthetics, despite their transformative capabilities, encounter challenges in terms of cost and accessibility. Not everyone has the means to afford these cutting-edge technologies, limiting their benefits to a select few. Additionally, the complexity of these devices requires ongoing maintenance and technical expertise, adding another layer of consideration and potential drawbacks.

Automation in pharmacies and laboratories, while streamlining processes, raises concerns about the displacement of human workers. Critics argue that the advantages in efficiency and accuracy come at the cost of job losses. Moreover, the complete reliance on automation introduces the potential for system failures, such as medication dispensing errors or technical glitches in laboratory testing, which could have significant repercussions on patient safety.

As the world of robotics in health care continues to evolve, stakeholders grapple with the balance between the advantages and disadvantages. It has become clear that while these technologies hold immense promise, they are not without their complexities and ethical considerations. Striking the right balance between technological advancements and human-centered care remains an ongoing pursuit, one that will shape the future of health care in remarkable ways.

Remote Monitoring: Key Innovators and the Technological Advancements Shaping Health Care

Remote Monitoring

Remote monitoring is the use of technology to monitor and track an individual's health status or medical condition from a distance. This may include devices that collect and transmit data, such as heart rate, blood pressure, or glucose levels, to a health care provider for analysis and treatment.

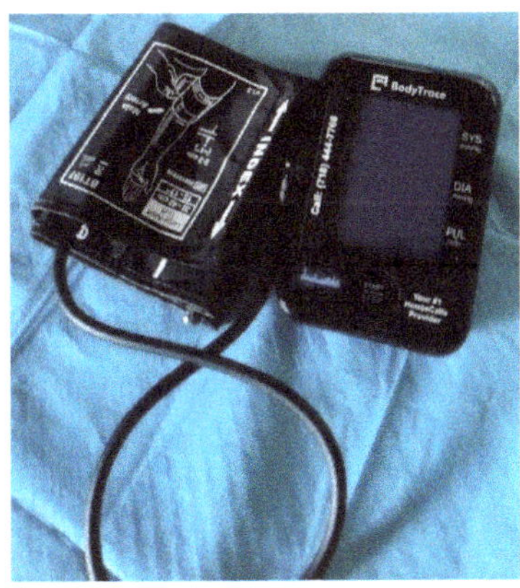

FIGURE 2.1 Remote blood pressure monitoring.

Major Contributors to Remote Monitoring

Several pioneers and key contributors have played significant roles in the development and advancement of remote monitoring. Here are a few notable figures:

- *Nikola Tesla (1856–1943)*: Tesla, a renowned inventor and electrical engineer, made substantial contributions to the field of remote communication. His work on wireless power transmission and radio technology laid the foundation for long-distance communication, which ultimately enabled remote monitoring.

- *Clarence F. Hansell (1901–1990)*: Hansell is often considered the father of remote sensing. He conducted extensive research on aerial photography and developed methods to collect and interpret data from remote locations. His work contributed to the early development of remote monitoring techniques.
- *David J. Bradley (1960s)*: Bradley is known for his contributions to the development of supervisory control and data acquisition (SCADA) systems. In the late 1960s, he pioneered the concept of real-time remote monitoring and control of industrial processes through the use of computers and communication networks. His work led to the widespread adoption of SCADA systems in industrial applications.
- *Theodore Paraskevakos (1968–1970)*: Paraskevakos, a Greek-American engineer, is credited with inventing the concept of the first wearable device with remote monitoring capabilities. In the 1970s, he developed a wearable device called the Electronic Man, which included sensors to monitor various physiological parameters. This invention laid the groundwork for modern wearable technology and remote patient monitoring.
- *Steve Mann (1978–1993)*: Mann, a researcher and inventor, has made significant contributions to the field of wearable computing and AR. His work in the 1980s and 1990s involved the development of wearable cameras and sensor systems, which contributed to the advancement of remote monitoring technologies.
- *Kevin Ashton (1999)*: Ashton, a British technologist, is often credited with coining the term *Internet of Things* (IoT). He played a crucial role in promoting the concept of interconnected devices and their potential for remote monitoring and data collection. Ashton's ideas laid the foundation for the rapid growth of IoT and its applications in remote monitoring.

These are just a few notable pioneers in the field of remote monitoring. There are many more researchers, engineers, and inventors who have contributed to the development and evolution of remote monitoring systems and technologies over time.

Remote Monitoring in Health Care: Enhancing Access, Outcomes, and Patient Engagement

Remote monitoring in health care is a practice that allows health care providers to monitor patients' health conditions from a distance. It utilizes technology to collect and transmit relevant health data to health care professionals, enabling them to assess patients' well-being and provide appropriate care (Martin, 2017). This approach eliminates the need for in-person visits and enables continuous monitoring, leading to improved patient outcomes and increased access to care.

At its core, remote monitoring involves the use of various devices and sensors that collect patients' vital signs, such as heart rate, blood pressure, blood glucose levels, oxygen saturation, and more. These devices can be wearable, like fitness trackers or smartwatches, or nonwearable, such as wireless blood pressure cuffs or glucose monitors.

The collected data is securely transmitted to health care providers through digital platforms, such as online portals or mobile applications. These platforms often integrate with EHR systems, allowing seamless access to patients' medical histories. Health care professionals can review the data remotely, analyze trends, and identify any abnormalities or changes that require attention.

Remote monitoring offers numerous benefits. It enables early detection of health issues, as changes in vital signs can be detected promptly. This allows health care providers to intervene quickly, preventing complications and reducing hospitalizations. Remote monitoring is particularly useful for patients with chronic conditions, as it provides continuous oversight of their health status and helps ensure adherence to treatment plans.

Furthermore, remote monitoring promotes patient engagement and empowerment. Patients have access to their own health data and can actively participate in their care. They can better understand their conditions, track progress, and make informed decisions about their lifestyles and treatments. This involvement often leads to improved self-management and overall health outcomes.

Advanced technologies, such as AI and ML, are also being integrated into remote monitoring systems. These technologies can analyze large datasets, identify patterns, and provide personalized insights and recommendations to both patients and health care providers. This helps in early identification of potential risks and enables tailored interventions.

Remote monitoring has the potential to transform health care delivery by increasing efficiency, reducing costs, and enhancing patient experiences. It allows health care providers to extend their reach beyond traditional care settings and overcome geographical barriers. Patients, especially those in remote or underserved areas, can benefit from timely interventions and improved access to specialized care.

Overall, remote monitoring in health care is a powerful tool that leverages technology to bring health care closer to patients. It enhances patient–provider communication, empowers individuals to take charge of their health, and contributes to a more patient-centered approach to care delivery.

Advantages of Remote Monitoring

In the realm of modern health care, the implementation of remote monitoring systems brought about both advantages and disadvantages, shaping the landscape of patient care:

- *Enhanced patient outcomes*: With remote monitoring systems, health care providers can keep a constant watch over patients' vital signs and health parameters without requiring their physical presence. This enables early detection of abnormalities, allowing for timely interventions and improved patient outcomes. Patients no longer need to be confined to hospital beds but can recover in familiar surroundings while still receiving quality care.
- *Increased efficiency and resource optimization*: In a bustling hospital, every second counts. Remote monitoring systems revolutionized the workflow by enabling health care professionals to monitor multiple patients simultaneously. Rather than being physically present in each patient's room, nurses and doctors can access real-time data from a centralized

location. This streamlined approach saves valuable time, allowing medical personnel to focus on critical tasks while still providing attentive care. Furthermore, remote monitoring reduces the need for frequent physical check-ups, optimizing resources and health care personnel allocation.

- *Cost-effectiveness and accessibility*: A major advantage of remote monitoring is its potential to lower health care costs and improve accessibility. By reducing the need for frequent hospital visits or extended stays, patients experience financial relief, and the burden of transportation or accommodation expenses is alleviated. Additionally, remote monitoring can extend health care services to underserved areas, where access to specialized care might be limited. This technology bridges the gap and allows health care providers to remotely monitor patients in remote regions, increasing access to quality care.

Disadvantages of Remote Monitoring

While remote monitoring has revolutionized health care with its numerous benefits, it also presents several challenges and limitations that impact its effectiveness and accessibility. These drawbacks highlight the complexities of integrating technology into patient care and the need for ongoing improvements:

- *Technological limitations and reliability*: As with any technological advancement, remote monitoring systems are not without their challenges. Dependence on technology introduces the risk of technical failures or malfunctions. Power outages, network disruptions, or software glitches could potentially interrupt the flow of vital data, causing delays in patient care. Ensuring system reliability and having backup mechanisms become paramount to mitigate these risks and maintain the continuity of monitoring services.
- *Potential data overload and interpretation challenges*: The vast amount of data generated by remote monitoring systems presents both a blessing and a curse. Health care professionals face the challenge of sifting through copious amounts of data, interpreting the information accurately, and prioritizing

critical alerts. The risk of information overload and the potential for overlooking important signals amid the noise requires careful attention. Developing effective algorithms and decision support systems become crucial to assist health care providers in navigating the sea of data and deriving meaningful insights.

- *Loss of personal connection and human touch*: In the pursuit of efficiency and remote care, some patients and health care providers feel a sense of detachment. The absence of physical presence and direct human interaction leaves a void that technology can't fully fill. Patients miss the comforting touch of a nurse's hand or the empathetic support of a caregiver at their bedside. Health care providers also experience a loss of connection with their patients, finding it challenging to build rapport and establish trust solely through virtual means. Striking a balance between technological advancements and preserving the human touch remains a crucial consideration.

In the realm of remote monitoring, the advantages and disadvantages intertwine, offering opportunities for improved patient care, workflow efficiency, and cost-effectiveness. However, challenges related to technology reliability, data interpretation, and the human aspect reminds health care professionals of the importance of maintaining a delicate equilibrium between technology and compassionate care.

Biometrics Authentication and Health Care

Biometrics refers to the measurement and analysis of unique physical or behavioral characteristics of individuals. It involves the use of advanced technologies to identify, authenticate, and verify the identity of individuals based on their distinct features. Common biometric characteristics include fingerprints, iris or retinal patterns, facial features, voice patterns, and even DNA.

The field of health care has been significantly impacted by the emergence of biometrics, which refers to the unique physical or behavioral attributes that distinguish individuals. In this context, biometrics plays a pivotal role in ensuring precise patient identification and enhancing health care delivery.

Traditionally, patient identification relied on methods such as identification cards or manual recordkeeping, which are prone to errors and inefficiencies. However, biometrics has introduced a more accurate and streamlined approach. By capturing and analyzing an individual's distinct physiological or behavioral traits like fingerprints, iris patterns, facial features, voice patterns, or gait, biometrics establishes a secure and reliable digital identity for each patient.

In the context of health care facilities, the integration of biometrics becomes evident from the moment a patient enters the premises. Instead of enduring cumbersome paperwork or presenting identification documents, patients can be swiftly identified using biometric data. High-tech sensors or cameras capture this data, which is then matched against the patient's EHR to ensure accurate identification without the need for manual intervention.

Moreover, biometrics extends beyond patient identification and significantly impacts the quality of care provided. Consider a scenario when a health care provider needs access to a patient's medical history to make informed decisions. With biometric authentication, such as fingerprint or iris scanning, health care providers can securely access a patient's EHR, granting them immediate access to crucial information like medical history, previous diagnoses, medications, and allergies. This streamlined access enables health care professionals to provide more personalized and well-informed care, saving time and enhancing patient outcomes.

Biometrics also addresses challenges related to medication management and safety. By leveraging biometric technology, such as fingerprint recognition on smart pill bottles, health care providers can ensure that the right patient is taking the correct medication at the appropriate time. This mitigates the risks associated with medication errors and enhances treatment adherence, ultimately improving patient safety and therapeutic outcomes.

Furthermore, biometrics finds utility in remote patient monitoring. Wearable devices equipped with biometric sensors enable continuous monitoring of vital signs like heart rate, blood pressure, and blood glucose levels. These devices transmit real-time data to health care providers, allowing them to remotely monitor patients' health status and intervene promptly if necessary. By facilitating remote monitoring, biometrics reduces the burden on health care facilities, enhances patient convenience, and improves overall health care delivery.

The integration of biometrics in health care has tremendous potential to revolutionize the industry. By optimizing patient identification, improving access to medical records, streamlining administrative processes, enhancing medication management, and enabling remote monitoring, biometrics strengthens the efficiency and effectiveness of health care services. This technological advancement holds the promise of improving patient outcomes, optimizing resource allocation, and transforming the health care experience as we know it.

By harnessing the power of biometrics and leveraging advanced informatics technologies, health care providers can deliver personalized, efficient, and data-driven care, leading to improved patient outcomes and a transformative health care experience.

Advantages of Biometrics in Health Care

The integration of biometrics in health care has introduced a range of advantages that enhance security, accuracy, and patient safety. By leveraging unique biological identifiers, biometric systems improve various aspects of health care operations, from patient identification to data protection and fraud prevention. Some key benefits include:

- Biometric authentication can be used to accurately identify patients, ensuring that the right medical records and treatments are assigned to the correct individuals. This helps prevent errors in diagnosis, treatment, and medication administration.
- Biometric systems can be employed to control access to secure areas within health care facilities, such as restricted wards, medication storage areas, and laboratories. This ensures that only authorized personnel can enter sensitive areas, improving security and safeguarding patient privacy.

- Biometric authentication can enhance the security of EHRs by adding an extra layer of protection. By using biometrics to authenticate health care providers, unauthorized access to patient data can be minimized, reducing the risk of data breaches and ensuring patient confidentiality.
- Biometric systems can be utilized to ensure accurate medication administration. By linking a patient's biometric data to their prescribed medications, health care providers can verify the identity of patients before administering medications, reducing the possibility of medication errors.
- Biometric sensors can be used to monitor patients' vital signs and physiological parameters, such as heart rate, blood pressure, and oxygen saturation. This real-time data can assist health care providers in detecting abnormalities or warning signs, allowing for early intervention and improved patient care.
- Biometrics can help prevent health care fraud by accurately verifying the identity of patients and providers. This can minimize instances of identity theft, insurance fraud, and duplicate records, leading to cost savings for health care organizations and insurers.

Disadvantages of Biometrics in Health Care

While biometrics offer many advantages in health care, they are not without their challenges. Issues like accuracy, privacy concerns, and system compatibility can create hurdles in their implementation. Some potential drawbacks include:

- While technological advancements have improved the accuracy of biometric systems, there will always be a margin of error. Factors such as changes in physical appearance, injuries, or environmental conditions can still impact the accuracy of biometric measurements, resulting in false positives or false negatives.
- Biometric data is inherently personal and unique to individuals. Once collected, it can be challenging to completely eliminate privacy concerns. Even with robust security measures, there is always a risk of unauthorized access, identity theft, or misuse of biometric data.

- Biometric systems raise ethical questions about consent, data ownership, and potential misuse. Although compliance with data protection laws and regulations can address some concerns, there may still be ethical dilemmas regarding the collection, storage, and use of biometric data.
- Biometric technologies in health care may lack standardized protocols across different systems or vendors. This lack of standardization can lead to compatibility issues and complexities during integration, making it difficult to achieve seamless interoperability.

While these disadvantages cannot be completely eliminated, health care organizations can take measures to minimize their impact and address them as effectively as possible through strict security protocols, transparency, informed consent, and compliance with relevant laws and regulations.

Networks

Networks are intricate systems that connect devices or computers, enabling the smooth exchange of information and data. In the context of health care, these networks play a crucial role in fostering communication and collaboration among health care providers. Additionally, they are utilized for effectively managing and sharing patient data and medical records.

Importance of Networks in Health Care

Networks play a vital role in health care by enabling seamless communication and collaboration among health care professionals. Through network connections, health care teams can share critical information, such as patient conditions, treatment plans, and test results, in real time. This promotes effective decision-making, enhances patient care coordination, and ultimately leads to improved patient outcomes.

In addition to communication, networks provide health care providers with access to a wide range of medical resources and knowledge. Through network connectivity, health care professionals can access online medical databases, research articles, medical journals, and educational materials. This access to a wealth of information helps them stay up-to-date with the latest advancements in their fields, make evidence-based decisions, and provide high-quality care to patients.

Networks have also revolutionized health care delivery through telemedicine and remote monitoring services. Patients can now connect with health care professionals remotely through network-enabled platforms, allowing for virtual consultations, diagnosis, and treatment. Networks also facilitate remote monitoring of patients' health conditions through wearable devices, IoT-enabled medical equipment, and home monitoring systems. This real-time monitoring allows health care providers to detect any anomalies and intervene promptly, even from a distance.

Efficient data management is another crucial aspect facilitated by networks in health care. EHRs can be accessed, updated, and shared securely across health care facilities within the network. This ensures that health care providers have instant access to comprehensive patient information, reducing errors, eliminating duplication, improving care coordination, and enhancing patient safety.

Moreover, networks contribute to medical research and advancements by facilitating the sharing and analysis of vast amounts of health care data. By connecting different health care organizations and research institutions, networks enable the pooling of data from various sources, resulting in larger and more diverse datasets. Researchers can then analyze this aggregated data to identify trends, patterns, and insights that inform evidence-based practices, clinical trials, and health care policies.

Different types of networks are used in health care to facilitate communication, data sharing, and collaboration among health care providers. These networks include local area networks (LANs) within individual health care facilities, wide area networks (WANs) that connect multiple health care sites, virtual private networks (VPNs) for secure remote access, and HIEs that enable interoperability between different health care organizations.

In summary, networks have transformed the health care landscape by connecting health care providers, improving communication and collaboration, providing access to medical resources, supporting telemedicine and remote monitoring, facilitating efficient data management, and driving medical research and innovation. These advancements have had a profound impact on patient care, leading to improved outcomes and enhanced health care delivery overall.

Summary

This chapter equips health professionals with the necessary processes, principles, and concepts to make meaningful use of the technology and systems presented. By understanding and applying algorithms, they can effectively capture patterns, trends, and insights to improve medical diagnoses, treatments, and patient care in telemedicine and remote consultations. Through the principles of empowerment and self-care, health professionals can guide patients to manage their health using self-manager devices and resources, thereby reducing health care costs. They learn to harness the power of robotics and automation, incorporating these concepts into surgical precision, rehabilitation, and daily living activities to optimize health care delivery and decrease expenses. The principles of real-time monitoring and remote access enable health professionals to improve health care services' accessibility and efficiency, while the concept of personalized health management plans ensures targeted interventions and prevention strategies for chronic conditions. With a focus on biometric authentication and privacy principles, health professionals ensure patient security while utilizing biometric technology to monitor health indicators and analyze population health trends. By embracing communication and collaboration principles, they leverage secure networks and information exchange systems to seamlessly access and share patient data and medical records, automating administrative tasks to enhance efficiency and cost-effectiveness. By employing these principles, concepts, and processes, health professionals can effectively make meaningful use of the technology and systems presented in this chapter, contributing to the advancement of health care quality and improved patient outcomes.

Chapter Review Questions

Directions: Consider what you learned in this chapter as you respond to the health care scenario and questions.

Health Care Scenario: Transforming Patient Care

Dr. Smith, a primary care physician, has recently integrated various technological advancements into her practice to improve patient care. She uses algorithms to analyze patient data and provide accurate diagnoses and treatment plans. Her patients use self-management devices to monitor their health, which has increased their engagement and reduced visits to the clinic. Dr. Smith has also introduced robotic-assisted surgeries for certain procedures, resulting in quicker recovery times for her patients.

To monitor chronic conditions in real time, Dr. Smith employs remote monitoring technology, allowing her to provide timely interventions and reduce hospitalizations. She emphasizes healthy aging by recommending personalized health management plans, which have helped many of her elderly patients delay the onset of chronic conditions.

To ensure patient data security, Dr. Smith uses biometric authentication methods. She also uses secure networks for efficient communication and collaboration with other health care providers, improving the overall efficiency of her practice.

Multiple-Choice Questions

1. Which specific aspect of algorithm application in Dr. Smith's practice contributes most significantly to enhanced patient outcomes in telemedicine?
   a. Standardization of medical records
   b. Personalized interventions based on data patterns and trends
   c. General patient education resources
   d. Automated billing processes

2. In what way do self-management devices contribute to the reduction of health care costs in Dr. Smith's practice?
   a. By eliminating the need for medical professionals
   b. Through early detection and management of health issues
   c. By reducing the production of medical devices
   d. Through the use of generic medication recommendations
3. What is a potential ethical consideration associated with the use of robotic-assisted surgeries in Dr. Smith's practice?
   a. The high cost of robotic systems
   b. The potential loss of surgical jobs
   c. Ensuring informed consent and managing patient expectations
   d. Increased need for postoperative care
4. How does real-time remote monitoring technology enhance the management of chronic conditions?
   a. By increasing the number of in-person consultations
   b. Through the provision of immediate feedback and intervention capabilities
   c. By eliminating the need for routine medical tests
   d. Through the use of standardized treatment protocols
5. Which key factor is most critical in promoting healthy aging through personalized health management plans?
   a. Standardized health education programs
   b. Individualized lifestyle recommendations based on patient data
   c. Increased reliance on medication
   d. Group therapy sessions
6. What is a primary advantage of using biometric authentication for patient data security in Dr. Smith's practice?
   a. It simplifies the login process for health care providers.
   b. It eliminates the need for physical security measures.

   c. It enhances the accuracy and reliability of patient identity verification.
   d. It replaces the need for electronic health records.

7. How does the use of secure networks and information exchange systems improve health care provider collaboration in Dr. Smith's practice?

   a. By allowing for the anonymous sharing of patient data
   b. By enabling real-time updates and access to patient records across different locations
   c. By reducing the need for face-to-face meetings
   d. By standardizing all medical treatments

Answer Key

1. (b) Personalized interventions based on data patterns and trends
2. (b) Through early detection and management of health issues
3. (c) Ensuring informed consent and managing patient expectations
4. (b) Through the provision of immediate feedback and intervention capabilities
5. (b) Individualized lifestyle recommendations based on patient data
6. (c) It enhances the accuracy and reliability of patient identity verification.
7. (b) By enabling real-time updates and access to patient records across different location

References

Ibn, R., Probst, P., Sims, J., Zirngibl, H., Bäuerle, T., Waldherr, C., & Radermacher, K. (2017). Fully automated, highly accurate segmentation of target volumes for radiotherapy of breast cancer. *Medical Physics*, *44*(2), 464–478.

Martin, R. C. (2017). Nikola Tesla (1856–1943): The mind behind the master of lighting. *Footnotes: A Journal of History*, *1*, 134–143.

Perez, M. V., Mahaffey, K. W., Hedlin, H., Rumsfeld, J. S., Garcia, A., Ferris, T., & Olgin, J. E. (2019). Large-scale assessment of a smartwatch to identify atrial fibrillation. *New England Journal of Medicine, 381*(20), 1909–1917.

Roguin, A. (2006). René-Théophile-Hyacinthe Laënnec (1781–1826): The man behind the stethoscope. *Clinical Medicine & Research, 4*(3), 230–235. https://doi.org/10.3121/cmr.4.3.230

Sittig, D. F., Ash, J. S., & Ledley, R. S. (2006). The story behind the development of the first whole-body computerized tomography scanner as told by Robert S. Ledley. *Journal of the American Medical Informatics Association, 13*(5), 465–469. https://doi.org/10.1197/jamia.M2127

West, J. B. (2008). Ibn al-Nafis, the pulmonary circulation, and the Islamic Golden Age. *Journal of Applied Physiology, 105*(6), 1877–1880. https://doi.org/10.1152/japplphysiol.91171.2008

Figure Credits

Chapter 3

Digital Tools in Health Programs

Strategies, Tactical Planning, and Logic Modeling

Introduction

The purpose of Chapter 3 is to delve into the strategies and tactical planning required for effectively using digital tools within health-related programs. This chapter aims to equip health informatics students with the necessary knowledge and skills to strategically plan and implement HIS and health information technology (HIT). By focusing on usability and leveraging technology, the chapter demonstrates how to enhance patient care, improve health care system accessibility, and optimize overall health care outcomes. The Health Guardian for Longevity Program (HGFLP) serves as a practical example, illustrating how strategic planning and digital tools can be employed to achieve positive health care results (Pemberton, 2021).

Chapter 3 is significant because it highlights the critical role of strategic and tactical planning in the successful implementation and utilization of HIS and HIT. It emphasizes the importance of understanding the symbiotic relationship between these planning approaches to pave the way for effective health informatics practices. By examining the intricacies of each planning component, the chapter provides a comprehensive understanding of how to align strategic planning with an organization's mission and vision, ultimately improving health care delivery and patient care. The insights gained from this chapter are crucial for health care professionals aiming to maximize outcomes and enhance the efficiency of systems through well-structured planning and effective use of digital tools.

By examining the implementation and outcomes of the HGFLP, readers will gain practical insights into how digital tools can be effectively employed in health-related programs to achieve positive results (Pemberton, 2017).

We'll break down strategic and tactical planning step by step, examining their individual components to see how they connect and contribute to the success of HIS and HIT initiatives. This focused approach provides valuable insights into creating, refining, and optimizing the planning process in health care organizations. Let's begin by exploring the key aspects of strategic planning and how it aligns with an organization's mission and vision.

Objectives That Lead to Outcomes

We have detailed specific goals and the expected outcomes. The following table aligns these key objectives with their corresponding outcomes, offering a clear and comprehensive understanding of what learners should achieve and comprehend upon completion. This alignment ensures that each objective is paired with a tangible and measurable outcome, thereby enhancing the overall learning experience. By presenting the objectives alongside their connected outcomes in a clear and structured manner, the table highlights the intended impacts of each initiative.

Objective	Outcome
Define and differentiate between strategic planning and tactical planning in HIS and HIT.	Clearly articulate the differences between strategic and tactical planning in HIS and HIT.
Identify the steps involved in strategic and tactical planning for the effective use of digital tools in a health-related program.	Understand the step-by-step process for planning and implementing digital tools in health care programs.

Analyze and assess problems or challenges within a health-related program to determine their impact on the target population and health care outcomes.	Identify and evaluate problems within health programs, understanding their effects on population health and program outcomes.
Develop a clear and well-justified rationale for implementing digital tools in a health-related program, highlighting the potential benefits and outcomes.	Justify the use of digital tools in health programs, outlining expected advantages and impact on health outcomes.
Design appropriate planning strategies and interventions to address identified problems and improve the health-related program.	Create effective planning strategies and interventions to solve identified issues and enhance program performance.
Evaluate and select automated tools and digital applications that support strategic and tactical planning processes.	Assess and choose suitable digital tools and applications that enhance planning processes in health care programs.

Key Terms

Directions: Before reading, please look at this list of key terms that will he used in this chapter. If any term is unfamiliar, please see the glossary at the end of the book.

algorithms
automated tools
conceptualization
data analysis
data collection
decision-making processes
digital applications
digital tools
evaluation
forecasting
health care outcomes
health informatics
Health Information systems (HIS)
health information technology (HIT)
health-related program
logic model
monitoring
optimization
patient care
planning strategies
problem identification
rationale development
resource allocation
strategic planning
tactical planning
target population

Strategic and Tactical Planning in HIS and HIT

In the dynamic world of health care, effective management of HIS and HIT is crucial for organizations to deliver optimal patient care and achieve their strategic objectives. Two critical components of this management are strategic planning and tactical planning. Strategic planning involves envisioning long-term goals and aligning technology initiatives with the organization's mission, while tactical planning focuses on the execution of specific actions to realize those strategic objectives. By establishing a clear flow between strategic and tactical planning in HIS and HIT, health care organizations can ensure that technology and information systems are utilized efficiently, leading to improved patient care and effective health care management.

Strategic Planning

Strategic planning involves formulating long-term goals and defining the overall direction of an organization's information systems and technology initiatives. It focuses on setting broad objectives and goals that align with the organization's mission and strategic objectives. In the realm of HIS and HIT, strategic planning typically encompasses a multiyear timeframe and involves high-level decision-making. It is concerned with identifying key priorities and assessing available resources and risks to achieve the organization's desired outcomes. In addition, strategic planning in HIS and HIT involves considering the organization's overall needs, technological advancements, regulatory requirements, and industry trends. Once the strategic plan is established, it needs to align with the organization's broader mission and vision. This ensures that the use of HIS and HIT contributes directly to achieving the organization's overall purpose. The outcomes of strategic planning guide the development and implementation of tactical plans. Here are the strategic planning steps:

1. *Define goals and objectives*: Clearly articulate the overall goals and objectives of the health-related program. Identify what you want to achieve through the use of digital tools, such as improving patient outcomes, enhancing efficiency, or increasing access to health care services.

2. *Conduct needs assessment*: Assess the specific needs and requirements of the program. Identify the areas in which digital tools can address challenges or provide solutions. This may involve evaluating existing systems, gathering feedback from stakeholders, and analyzing data.
3. *Identify digital tools and technologies*: Research and identify the digital tools and technologies that align with the program's goals and can address the identified needs. Consider tools such as EHRs, telemedicine platforms, data analytics tools, mobile applications, or wearable devices.
4. *Develop an implementation strategy*: Create a detailed plan for implementing the selected digital tools. This includes determining the timeline, resource allocation, and key milestones. Consider factors such as budget, technical infrastructure requirements, training needs, and potential barriers to adoption.
5. *Establish governance and stakeholder engagement*: Define the governance structure for overseeing the use of digital tools in the program. Identify the key stakeholders, such as health care providers, IT staff, administrators, and patients, and involve them in decision-making processes and implementation planning.

Tactical Planning

Now that we've covered strategic planning, let's move on to the exciting world of tactical planning. Tactical planning is the process of translating the strategic goals and objectives established during strategic planning into specific action plans and activities. It involves shorter-term planning and focuses on the operational details necessary to execute the strategic initiatives effectively by breaking down the strategic goals into practical tasks for implementation. Tactical planning in HIS and HIT involves identifying specific projects, tasks, and timelines that contribute to the achievement of the strategic objectives. It takes into account the available resources, operational constraints, and specific requirements of different departments or functional areas within the organization. As related to resource allocation, tactical planning requires allocating the necessary resources, such as finances, skilled personnel, and technological support, to execute the identified initiatives successfully. Tactical planning also considers the potential impact of the planned activities on the organization's day-to-day operations and stakeholders. This ensures that the organization has the capacity to implement HIS and HIT projects effectively. Here are the steps for tactical planning:

1. *Define specific objectives*: Translate the strategic goals into specific, measurable objectives for the use of digital tools. These objectives should be actionable, time-bound, and aligned with the overall program goals.
2. *Assess resource requirements*: Determine the resources needed for implementing and maintaining the digital tools. This includes financial resources, IT infrastructure, personnel, and training requirements. Assess the feasibility and availability of these resources.
3. *Develop an implementation plan*: Create a detailed plan that outlines the specific actions required to implement the digital tools. This includes tasks, responsibilities, timelines, and dependencies. Consider potential risks and develop contingency plans.
4. *Execute and monitor progress*: Execute the implementation plan, ensuring that tasks are completed according to the defined timeline. Monitor the progress regularly, track key performance indicators, and address any issues or challenges that arise.
5. *Evaluate and adjust*: Continuously evaluate the effectiveness and impact of the digital tools in achieving the program objectives. Collect feedback from users and stakeholders, analyze data and metrics, and make necessary adjustments to optimize the use of digital tools.
6. *Provide training and support*: Develop and deliver training programs to ensure that users are proficient in utilizing the digital tools effectively. Offer ongoing technical support and assistance to address any user issues or questions.

As you embark on this journey of organizational planning, gaining a clear grasp of the distinction between strategic and tactical planning is of utmost importance. It's crucial to understand the difference between strategic and tactical planning. These planning approaches play vital roles in achieving success for health care practices, businesses, and other ventures.

Imagine yourself as the team leader, shaping the future of your organization. In strategic planning, you hold the reins and set the ultimate goals and direction for your team. We'll explore various factors like market trends, customer needs, and competition to identify what makes your organization unique; we call this concept *differentiation*.

As we implement the HIS and HIT initiatives, we'll continuously monitor and evaluate their performance and impact on the organization's strategic objectives. We'll track key performance indicators (KPIs) to gauge success and pinpoint areas for improvement. The insights we gain from this process will feed back into our strategic planning, helping us refine and adjust our overall direction to adapt to changing health care needs effectively, as we get ready to move into tactical planning.

Remember, the flow between strategic and tactical planning is a continuous cycle of building and rebuilding. As our organization evolves and the health care landscape changes, our HIS and HIT planning must remain dynamic and forward-thinking to support our objectives effectively. This constant striving for improvement ensures that we optimize our information systems and technology infrastructure, leading to improved patient care and effective health care management.

As we move deeper into this world of organizational planning, keep in mind the significance of strategic thinking and how it shapes the future of our organization. Together, we'll make a difference and create a positive impact on health care practices.

Strategic and Tactical Differentiation

Differentiation is a significant concept in strategic planning. It's about finding and highlighting the special qualities that make your organization stand out from the crowd. It's not just about being different for the sake of it; it's about capitalizing on your strengths and capabilities to offer something valuable and distinct to your customers. Imagine your health informatics course as a cutting-edge medical facility, equipped with the latest technology and innovative tools. Once the strategic planning phase is complete, it's time to shift gears and move into tactical planning. This phase is when all the action happens, just like a medical team springing into action to provide top-notch patient care.

Tactical planning in your health informatics course is akin to implementing the carefully crafted strategies you've developed during the strategic planning phase. It's about breaking down those high-level objectives into smaller, manageable tasks for different teams or individuals, much like specialized medical professionals collaborating to deliver effective treatment to patients.

This is when differentiation comes into play again, but this time at a more detailed level. In tactical planning, you work on the specific steps to implement the unique features and advantages you've identified during strategic planning. Think of it as ensuring that every student knows their role and responsibilities, working in harmony to create a transformative learning experience that sets your health informatics program apart.

Just as a state-of-the-art medical facility attracts patients seeking the best care, your well-executed tactical planning will make your health informatics program stand out and attract eager students who are excited to learn from your program's unique and valuable offerings. During tactical planning, you'll fine-tune marketing strategies, optimize customer experiences, and enhance your products or services' unique aspects. By doing so, you reinforce your organization's distinctiveness and competitive edge in the market. It's like making sure your health team operates seamlessly, like a well-oiled machine, offering a digital journey that clients can't resist.

To recap, the journey from strategic to tactical planning is crucial for any organization. By understanding differentiation, you can move confidently toward success. Strategic planning provides the roadmap and identifies what makes your organization unique. Tactical planning ensures that you put those unique qualities into action, making your organization shine in the market. By combining these two planning approaches, you will successfully achieve your program objectives and stand out in the vast telehealth market, in which a host of business opportunities will prevail.

Differentiation in Strategic Planning

In the strategic planning phase, as the team leader, you take charge of setting the organization's ultimate goals and direction. The process involves careful analysis of various factors, including market trends, customer needs, and competition. This analysis is vital for identifying what makes the organization unique, which is precisely what differentiation is all about.

Differentiation, at the strategic level, means understanding and leveraging the organization's strengths, resources, and capabilities to create a distinct value proposition. It involves answering questions such as "What unique services can the organization offer to an elderly population? How can it stand out from other care providers in the market? What sets it apart and makes it the preferred choice for the community's needs?"

By focusing on differentiation during strategic planning, you ensure that the organization's vision aligns with its unique selling points, making it well-positioned to meet the specific demands and challenges of providing care to the elderly population, as in a case of a local hospital's closure, as an aspect of one scenario.

Differentiation in Tactical Planning

Once the strategic planning phase is complete, the focus shifts to tactical planning. In tactical planning, you break down the strategic goals into actionable steps and allocate resources to implement the defined strategy effectively.

Differentiation continues to play a vital role at the tactical level. It involves translating the identified uniqueness and competitive advantage into specific, practical actions. For example, if the organization's differentiation lies in personalized care plans, tactical planning would involve establishing procedures and training staff to develop and implement these individualized care approaches.

Tactical planning also ensures that day-to-day operations align with the organization's strategic vision and unique value proposition. This could involve marketing efforts to communicate the organization's distinct services, optimizing customer experiences to reflect the unique care approach, and fostering a culture of compassion and warmth among staff to reinforce the organization's differentiation. By seamlessly integrating differentiation into both planning levels, the organization can effectively navigate challenges and achieve its objectives while standing out in the competitive market. Figure 3.1 sheds light on strategic planning as broad and holistic, encompassing the overall direction, objectives, and resource allocation for the organization's HIS and HIT initiatives.

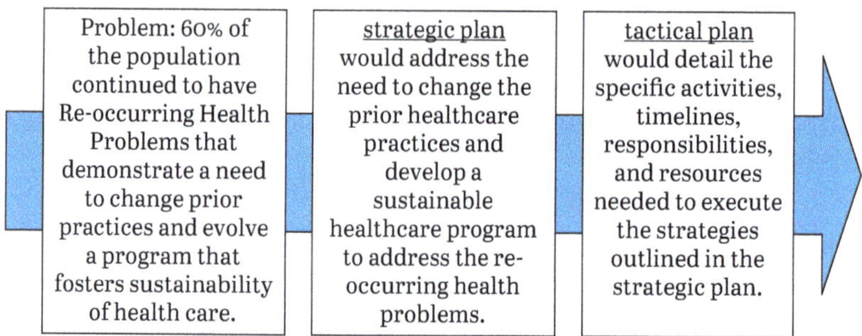

FIGURE 3.1 Planning process.

Tactical planning is more focused and operational, detailing specific actions, tasks, and timelines required to accomplish the strategic objectives. Remember that these steps in both strategic and tactical planning strategies provide a general framework, and the actual planning process may involve additional considerations based on the specific program and organization. Adapt and customize these steps to fit the unique needs and context of your health-related program and organization.

Analyzing Challenges and Leveraging Digital Tools for Informed Decision-Making in Health Care

In today's rapidly evolving health care landscape, optimizing health-related programs and leveraging digital tools in the planning process has become crucial. By analyzing and assessing program challenges, health informatics professionals gain valuable insights into the obstacles that exist within health-related programs. This process involves thoroughly understanding and evaluating issues such as limited resources or inefficiencies in service delivery. By comprehending these challenges and their implications on the target population and health care outcomes, informed decisions can be made to drive improvements in health care delivery and patient outcomes. This knowledge serves as a foundation for justifying the use of digital tools, designing effective interventions, evaluating algorithms, and applying acquired knowledge to real-world scenarios. Through these strategic approaches, health informatics plays a pivotal role in addressing program challenges and driving positive change in the health care landscape.

Once the challenges have been identified, conducting a comprehensive analysis of the target population becomes crucial. This analysis considers demographic, socioeconomic, and cultural factors that influence planning decisions. By understanding these elements, planners can develop programs that are tailored to the specific needs and preferences of the population, ensuring that interventions are culturally sensitive, accessible, and effective.

Harnessing the Power of Digital Tools

Advancing Health Care in the Digital Age

In the digital age, it is important to develop a clear and well-justified rationale for implementing digital tools in health-related programs. These tools offer potential benefits such as improved efficiency, enhanced data management, increased accessibility, and better patient engagement. By embracing digital solutions, health programs can unlock opportunities for innovation and improved health care delivery.

Designing appropriate planning strategies and interventions is the next step. Building on the analysis of challenges and target population, planners can develop interventions that directly address identified problems and improve the health-related program. Evidence-based practices and insights from health informatics guide the development of interventions that are effective, efficient, and tailored to the specific needs of the population.

To guide the implementation and evaluation of planned interventions, a logic model is created. This model outlines the inputs, processes, outputs, and outcomes of the interventions. It provides a structured framework for monitoring progress, assessing impact, and making informed adjustments to the program, ensuring alignment with goals and objectives throughout implementation.

Selecting the right automated tools and digital applications is crucial for effective planning processes. By evaluating available options, health informatics professionals can identify tools that support strategic and tactical planning. These tools streamline data analysis, enhance forecasting capabilities, and facilitate resource allocation, contributing to the program's overall success.

While automated tools offer numerous benefits, it's important to acknowledge and address the associated challenges. Data security, user training, and potential biases need to be considered. By understanding these benefits and challenges, health professionals can make informed decisions and mitigate potential risks during the planning phase.

Illustration of a Logic Model for Case 1

Ms. C. was hospitalized after suffering a heart attack and is currently being discharged. In addition to the usual prescriptions and post-discharge instructions, Ms. C. has been enrolled in the HGFLP and equipped with the tools needed to participate.

TABLE 3.1 Logic Model for the Home-based HGFLP

Inputs	Activities	Outputs	Outcomes
Ms. C.'s health data and assessment results HGFLP Loaner laptop with webcam, built-in speakers, and internet access Smartphone with 5G capability and preloaded remote monitoring functions and interactive applications Access code for Ms. C. to access her private page on the program's website	Enrollment of Ms. C. into the HGFLP Provision of necessary tools and devices (laptop, smartphone) Set up Ms. C.'s home with the provided equipment Create a personalized private page on the program's website for Ms. C. Provide prescriptions and post-discharge instructions Train Ms. C. on how to use the laptop, smartphone, and program features Monitor Ms. C.'s health remotely using the program's functions and applications Regularly update and maintain the program's website and features	Ms. C.'s participation in the HGFLP Improved access to health care and remote monitoring for Ms. C. Increased knowledge and understanding of Ms. C. about her health condition and self-management Timely and accurate transmission of health data from Ms. C.'s devices to health care providers Regular communication and feedback between Ms. C. and health care providers Improved adherence to prescriptions and post-discharge instructions Enhanced engagement and empowerment of Ms. C. in her own health care journey	Improved health outcomes for Ms. C., including better management of her heart condition. Increased patient satisfaction and perceived value of the HGFLP. Potential positive impact on other patient–client health outcomes globally. Enhanced personal connection and sense of specialness among participants in the program. Increased awareness and adoption of remote monitoring technologies in health care.

Note: This logic model is based on the information provided and is a generalized representation. The specific details and outcomes may vary depending on the actual implementation and effectiveness of the program.

Enhancing Planning Processes and Decision-Making Through Algorithmic Optimization in Health Programs

Algorithms play a vital role in optimizing planning processes within health-related programs. They enable data analysis, forecasting, and resource allocation, leading to more accurate and efficient decision-making. Leveraging algorithms allows planners to identify trends, predict outcomes, and allocate resources effectively, enhancing the overall planning process.

The knowledge gained through strategic and tactical planning, along with digital tools, can be applied to real-world scenarios in health informatics. By translating theoretical concepts into practical applications, health professionals can drive meaningful improvements in health care outcomes. By analyzing challenges, considering the target population, justifying digital tools, designing interventions, evaluating algorithms, and applying knowledge to real-world scenarios, health informatics can revolutionize the planning and implementation of health-related programs, ultimately leading to improved health care outcomes for the population.

Modeling Strategic and Tactical Planning in the HGFLP

A Practical Implementation of Health Care Transformation

The HGFLP serves as a comprehensive web-based program, providing readers with a deep understanding of the discussed concepts and components (Pemberton, 2017). This program exemplifies the principles and strategic planning emphasized throughout, showcasing the transformative potential of HIT in health care. By exploring the program's intricacies, readers can witness firsthand the practical implementation of these ideas.

Exploring Practical Implementation in HIT

Through a thorough examination of the HGFLP, individuals embark on a journey of practical implementation. This immersive experience offers insights into the program's methodologies, strategies, and components. Leveraging advanced technologies, such as user-friendly interfaces and seamless data flow integration, the program demonstrates how digital systems can revolutionize health care delivery and management. This exploration deepens readers' comprehension of the vital role HIT plays in improving health outcomes.

Strategic Planning

The HGFLP begins with strategic planning, setting its overarching vision and objectives, including improving health outcomes and promoting longevity. This phase involves problem identification, extensive research, and data collection, forming the foundation for subsequent tactical planning (Pemberton, 2021). These strategic components provide a roadmap for decision-making, ensuring a solid groundwork for effective execution.

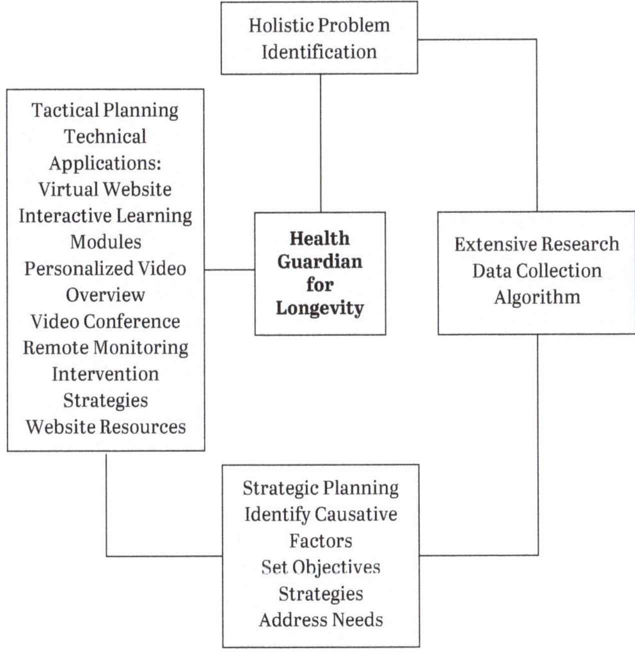

FIGURE 3.2 Health guardian taking center stage.

Tactical Planning

Taking center stage in the HGFLP, tactical planning focuses on the practical implementation of strategies outlined in the strategic plan. The program identifies specific actions, timelines, and resource allocations to enhance the usability of its HIS. User-friendly interfaces and innovative technologies are integrated, facilitating seamless data flow within the program's databases.

Bridging the Gap Between Vision and Execution

Through the alignment of tactical plans with the program's strategic goals, the HGFLP effectively bridges the gap between vision and execution. By translating broader objectives into tangible steps, the program optimizes the usability and effectiveness of its HIS. This reinforces commitment to promoting longevity and improving health outcomes, ensuring the successful realization of an organization's strategic vision.

Explanation of the Application to the HGFLP

The HGFLP is an illustration to understand how strategic and tactical planning contribute to the successful implementation of HIT. A step-by-step explanation is presented for the reader next.

Strategic Planning Step-by-Step

Step 1: Establishing Vision and Goals

The HGFLP begins with strategic planning, which involves defining the program's overarching vision and objectives. The primary goal may be to improve health care outcomes and patient satisfaction through the implementation of HIT solutions. During this stage, key stakeholders—including health care providers, administrators, and IT professionals—collaborate to set clear objectives, identify target populations, and outline the desired outcomes.

Step 2: Conducting Needs Assessment and Feasibility Analysis

To ensure a strong foundation, a thorough needs assessment is conducted to evaluate the current health care landscape, technological infrastructure, and patient demographics. This step helps determine existing gaps in care, resource availability, and potential challenges that may arise during implementation. A feasibility analysis is also carried out to assess whether the proposed HIT solutions can be effectively integrated into the current system and to identify any modifications needed for successful execution.

Step 3: Identifying Key Stakeholders and Resources

Successful strategic planning requires identifying the individuals and organizations that will play a crucial role in the program's development and execution. This includes securing necessary funding, forming partnerships with health care institutions, and ensuring IT support for seamless technology integration. By clarifying roles and responsibilities early on, the program can establish a strong collaborative framework that enhances efficiency and accountability.

Step 4: Developing a Strategic Road Map

Once the vision, goals, and resources are defined, a strategic road map is created to guide the program's implementation. This road map outlines specific steps, timelines, and milestones to ensure a smooth rollout. It includes plans for technology deployment, training programs for users, data monitoring strategies, and ongoing evaluation methods to measure the program's success. By providing a structured approach, the road map ensures that each phase of implementation aligns with the overall objectives.

Developing a HIT Strategy

Based on the strategic goals, the HGFLP formulates a HIT strategy that aligns with the desired outcomes. This involves determining the specific HIT solutions to be implemented and the expected benefits. For instance, the program might focus on implementing an EHR system to improve care coordination, reduce errors, and enhance data accessibility. The HIT strategy would outline the selection criteria, budgetary considerations, implementation timeline, and resource allocation required for the chosen HIT solution.

Tactical Development

Using the HGFLP as an illustration, tactical planning involves breaking down the overarching goals of the program into specific, actionable steps. For example, if the goal of the HGFLP is to reduce obesity rates in a community, tactical planning would involve determining the specific interventions and activities that will be implemented to achieve this goal. Tactical planning would address questions such as what resources are needed, which stakeholders will be involved, and how the interventions will be implemented. For instance, it might involve planning and organizing community health campaigns, developing educational materials, coordinating with local health care providers, and establishing partnerships with schools or fitness centers to promote physical activity and healthy eating habits.

Through tactical planning, the HGFLP would set specific objectives, define measurable outcomes, allocate resources effectively, and establish timelines for implementation. It would also involve considering potential barriers or challenges that may arise during the execution of the plan and developing contingency strategies to address them.

The role of tactical planning within the HGFLP is to bridge the gap between the broad strategic goals and the day-to-day operations. It provides a clear roadmap for executing the strategies and activities necessary to achieve desired outcomes. Tactical planning ensures that the program's efforts are focused, efficient, and aligned with the overall vision, maximizing the chances of success. Furthermore, tactical planning allows for ongoing monitoring and evaluation of the program's progress. By setting measurable objectives and defining specific indicators, the HGFLP can assess the effectiveness of its interventions, make necessary adjustments, and identify areas for improvement.

Tactical planning within a health-related program, such as the HGFLP, involves the detailed planning and execution of specific strategies and activities to achieve predefined goals. It ensures the effective implementation of interventions, proper allocation of resources, and the ability to monitor progress toward desired outcomes. Tactical planning is essential for translating strategic goals into actionable steps and maximizing the program's effectiveness in improving health outcomes. It also includes establishing KPIs and metrics to measure the progress and success of the HIT implementation. These KPIs could include improved patient record accuracy, reduced documentation time, or increased interoperability between health care systems.

Deployment and Operationalization of HIT Solutions

The HGFLP proceeds to implement the HIT solution as outlined in the tactical plan. This stage involves tasks such as configuring the EHR system; training end users, health care staff, and the community on its use; conducting user acceptance testing; and addressing any technical or operational challenges that arise during the implementation process. Regular communication and collaboration among stakeholders are vital to ensure smooth execution, troubleshoot issues promptly, and maintain alignment with the strategic goals.

Monitoring and Evaluation

Once the HIT solution is implemented, the HGFLP utilizes monitoring and evaluation mechanisms to assess its effectiveness. This involves measuring the defined KPIs, gathering feedback from end users, conducting research, and conducting usability assessments to identify areas of improvement.

Monitoring and evaluation allow those implementing the program to make data-driven decisions, refine processes, and enhance the HIT solution's performance throughout its deployment. This ongoing assessment ensures that the HGFLP is implemented in a systematic, well-coordinated manner and remains aligned with strategic objectives to achieve the desired outcomes.

Strategic and Tactical Planning for HIS Usability in HIT

The significance of strategic planning in HIS usability lies in how decision-makers use it to ensure that the design and implementation of HIS align with the needs and workflows of health care professionals and organizations. By incorporating strategic planning, usability considerations are integrated from the early stages of system development, leading to improved user experiences, enhanced efficiency, and increased patient safety.

Strategic planning also enables the identification of potential barriers and challenges in the usability of HIS, allowing for proactive measures to address these issues. It promotes collaboration among stakeholders, such as health care providers, IT professionals, and system users, fostering a shared vision and understanding of usability goals. This collaborative approach helps in aligning resources and efforts toward creating HIS that are user-friendly, intuitive, and supportive of efficient clinical workflows.

Additionally, strategic planning supports long-term sustainability and continuous improvement of HIS usability. By implementing an ongoing evaluation and feedback mechanism, organizations can monitor the effectiveness of usability interventions and identify areas for further enhancements. This iterative process ensures that HIS remains adaptable and responsive to changing user needs, technological advancements, and evolving health care requirements.

Strategic planning in the context of HIS usability is crucial for designing, implementing, and maintaining HIS that effectively support health care professionals and organizations. The Office of the National Coordinator for Health Information Technology (2020) report serves as an affirmation that the goals presented in this chapter will lead to the achievement of desirable outcomes. It also notes the following goals that conceptually align with the strategic and tactical plan presented in this chapter.

Goal 1: Expanding Access to Care and Optimizing Health Outcomes

Aligning the strategic and tactical plans with goal 1 demonstrates a commitment to leveraging HIT to improve access to care and enhance health outcomes. It highlights how the strategic plan incorporates telehealth solutions, interoperable systems, and patient engagement tools to ensure equitable access and personalized care for individuals.

Goal 2: Advancing Secure and Interoperable HIT Infrastructure

A secure and interoperable HIT infrastructure, which adopts standardized data formats, health information exchange networks, and cybersecurity measures, enables seamless data sharing while safeguarding patient privacy and protecting against potential threats.

Goal 3: Strengthening and Leveraging the HIT Workforce

The HGFLP leadership team's connection of the strategic plan with Goal 3 underscores a commitment to developing and empowering a skilled HIT workforce, as well as supporting patients as self-managers of care. This goal includes initiatives such as the creation of programs like HGFLP, training opportunities, professional development, and collaboration with educational institutions. These efforts aim to ensure a competent health informatics workforce capable of effectively implementing and maintaining HIT solutions.

Goal 4: Advancing Research, Scientific Knowledge, and Innovation

The strategic and tactical plan emphasizes advancing research, scientific knowledge, and innovation in HIT. By fostering collaboration among researchers, clinicians, and technology experts, we can drive the development and adoption of cutting-edge technologies and evidence-based practices that continuously improve health care delivery. Aligning these efforts with the four strategic goals ensures a comprehensive approach—expanding access to care, enhancing interoperability, investing in the workforce, and driving innovation.

To fully realize these objectives, planning must go beyond implementation. HIS need to be optimized to deliver meaningful benefits for health care professionals and organizations. The Office of the National Coordinator for Health Information Technology (2020) echoes these priorities, reinforcing the importance of intentional and forward-thinking decision-making in HIT.

By embracing a proactive planning mindset, we can enhance HIS usability, streamline workflows, and create a more adaptable, patient-centered health care system. Innovation and continuous improvement must remain at the forefront, ensuring that technology evolves to meet the changing needs of health care. Now is the time to take action—working together to build a smarter, more connected future.

To support these efforts, a range of digital tools can facilitate both strategic and tactical planning in health-related programs. These tools enhance collaboration, streamline data analysis, improve visualization, and strengthen decision-making. Let's explore some of the most effective options.

Sample Digital Tools for Planning in Health-Related Programs

Digital Tools for Effective Planning in Health Programs

Technology plays a vital role in streamlining the planning and management of health-related programs. Choosing the right digital tools can enhance organization, improve collaboration, and ensure efficient execution of tasks. Project management platforms such as Trello, Asana, and Microsoft Project offer structured solutions that help teams develop strategic plans, assign responsibilities, set deadlines, and track progress.

Each tool brings unique strengths that cater to different needs. Trello's simple, visual interface makes it an excellent choice for smaller teams or projects that require flexibility in task management. Asana, with its advanced features like task dependencies and portfolio management, is well-suited for large-scale health initiatives requiring more detailed oversight. Meanwhile, Microsoft Project provides powerful scheduling and resource management capabilities, making it an ideal option for complex programs that demand meticulous coordination.

Beyond basic task management, these platforms also support collaboration through file sharing, real-time communication, and integration with other health information systems. By leveraging these digital tools, health care teams can not only stay organized but also enhance efficiency, ensuring that initiatives are executed smoothly and effectively. Selecting the right tool depends on the specific needs of the program, the complexity of tasks, and the preferred working style of the team. With the right technology in place, planning health programs becomes a more streamlined and impactful process.

Sample Tools for Health Data Analysis, Communication, and Visualization

Data analytics and visualization tools like Tableau, Power BI, or Google Data Studio play a crucial role in planning by helping to analyze and visualize health data. By exploring trends, patterns, and insights from large datasets, these tools enable data-driven decision-making and identify strategic opportunities.

Geographic information systems (GIS) tools, such as ArcGIS or QGIS, are particularly useful for health planning with spatial data. These tools allow for mapping disease outbreaks, identifying vulnerable populations, and optimizing the allocation of health care resources based on geographic factors.

Communication and collaboration tools like Slack, Microsoft Teams, or Google Workspace facilitate effective communication and teamwork. They offer real-time messaging, file sharing, videoconferencing, and document collaboration features, enabling seamless coordination among team members involved in the planning process.

Mobile data collection tools, such as Open Data Kit (ODK), CommCare, or SurveyCTO, streamline data collection in the field. Health workers can collect data using mobile devices, whether online or offline, ensuring accuracy and timeliness while simplifying the data collection process.

Simulation and modeling tools like AnyLogic or MATLAB allow for the analysis of complex health systems. These tools assist in strategic planning by simulating the impact of different interventions, forecasting resource needs, and optimizing program designs before implementation.

EHR systems, including Epic, Cerner, or OpenMRS, offer a digital infrastructure for managing patient health records. By improving data accuracy, accessibility, and interoperability, EHR systems support better patient care and informed decision-making in planning.

When evaluating the usability and effectiveness of digital tools for planning, consider factors such as ease of use, compatibility with existing systems, features and functionality, scalability, data security and privacy, cost, and user feedback. These criteria will help you select the most suitable tools for your health-related program planning needs. By leveraging these digital tools and conducting a thorough evaluation, you can enhance the efficiency and effectiveness of planning in health-related programs, leading to improved outcomes and better allocation of resources.

SAMPLE OF APPLICATIONS YOU CAN USE TO CREATE YOUR OWN INTERACTIVE DASHBOARD

- *Qlik Sense*: Qlik Sense provides a free version called Qlik Sense Desktop, which allows you to create visually appealing dashboards using drag-and-drop functionality. It supports data integration from multiple sources.
- *Metabase*: Metabase is an open-source business intelligence tool that offers a free version. It enables you to create interactive dashboards and visualizations using simple SQL queries or a visual query builder.
- *Databox*: Databox offers a free plan that allows you to create dashboards by connecting to various data sources, including Google Analytics, social media platforms, and more. It provides prebuilt templates and customizable widgets.
- *Grafana*: Grafana is an open-source platform used for monitoring and data visualization. It offers a free version and allows you to create dynamic and customizable dashboards for visualizing time-series data.

These applications provide a range of features and capabilities for creating dashboards. You can explore their documentation, tutorials, and community support to get started with creating your own dashboard based on your specific needs and data sources.

These tools play a vital role in leveraging technology to support various aspects of health care management and decision-making. By harnessing the capabilities of digital applications, health care professionals can enhance efficiency, improve data analysis, and facilitate seamless communication, ultimately leading to better health care outcomes and patient care.

Summary

Chapter 3 provided a comprehensive look at the strategic and tactical planning required to effectively implement and optimize HIS. It outlined the structured approach needed to align HIT initiatives with key goals, including improving access to care, enhancing interoperability, strengthening the workforce, and fostering innovation. The chapter emphasized that successful planning goes beyond implementation—it requires continuous evaluation and adaptation to ensure that HIS solutions truly benefit health care professionals and patients.

A key takeaway was the role of digital tools in streamlining health program management. Platforms such as Trello, Asana, and Microsoft Project were explored as practical solutions for organizing tasks, improving collaboration, and tracking progress. These tools enhance efficiency in planning processes, ensuring that HIT initiatives are executed effectively.

Ultimately, the chapter reinforced the necessity of proactive decision-making and technological integration in HIT. By combining strategic foresight with the right tools, health care organizations can drive meaningful improvements, making systems more user-friendly, adaptable, and impactful in delivering quality care.

Chapter Review Questions

Directions: Consider what you learned in this chapter as you respond to the health care scenario and questions.

Health Care Scenario: The HGFLP

XYZ Health Clinic has recently launched the HGFLP. The program focuses on leveraging digital tools to improve usability, accessibility, and overall efficiency within the health care system. Health informatics students are involved in this program to gain practical insights and hands-on experience in strategic and tactical planning for HIS and HIT.

The purpose of this initiative is to delve into the strategies and tactical planning required for effectively using digital tools within health-related programs. By focusing on usability and leveraging technology, the HGFLP aims to demonstrate how to enhance patient care, improve health care system accessibility, and optimize overall health care outcomes.

Multiple-Choice Questions

1. How can strategic planning in the HGFLP ensure alignment with the clinic's mission to enhance patient care through digital tools?

    a. By prioritizing cost-cutting measures
    b. By focusing on expanding physical facilities
    c. By integrating digital tools to improve health care delivery
    d. By reducing staff training initiatives

2. In what way does tactical planning contribute to the successful implementation of HIS in the HGFLP?

    a. By increasing administrative overhead
    b. By scheduling regular IT upgrades
    c. By reducing patient interaction times
    d. By limiting access to patient data

3. How can the HGFLP effectively implement digital tools to improve patient care outcomes?

    a. By decreasing the use of technology in daily operations
    b. By involving health informatics students in strategic planning
    c. By delaying the adoption of HIT
    d. By increasing paperwork for health care professionals

4. What methods should XYZ Health Clinic employ to evaluate the effectiveness of the HGFLP?
    a. Ignoring patient feedback
    b. Conducting regular performance reviews and data analysis
    c. Limiting access to program outcomes
    d. Eliminating strategic goals
5. How can XYZ Health Clinic ensure continuous improvement in the implementation of digital tools within the HGFLP?
    a. By maintaining outdated technology
    b. By avoiding feedback from health care professionals
    c. By investing in ongoing training and technology updates
    d. By reducing patient access to medical records
6. What roles do health informatics students play in enhancing the effectiveness of the HGFLP? They enhance the effectiveness by
    a. avoiding participation in strategic planning
    b. focusing solely on theoretical concepts
    c. contributing practical insights and skills in HIS and HIT implementation
    d. ignoring advancements in health care technology

Answer Key

1. (c) By integrating digital tools to improve health care delivery
2. (b) By scheduling regular IT upgrades
3. (b) By involving health informatics students in strategic planning
4. (b) Conducting regular performance reviews and data analysis
5. (c) By investing in ongoing training and technology updates
6. (c) Contributing practical insights and skills in HIS and HIT implementation

References

Office of the National Coordinator for Health Information Technology. (2020, October). *2020–2025 federal health IT strategic plan*. https://www.healthit.gov/sites/default/files/page/2020-10/Federal%20Health%20IT%20Strategic%20Plan_2020_2025.pdf

Pemberton, F. (2017). A tailored approach is key: The Health Guardian for Longevity Program uses mobile technology to sustain healthy life behaviors. *COJ Nursing & Healthcare, 1*(1). https://doi.org/10.31031/COJNH.2017.01.000501

Pemberton, F. (2021). Village participants' perceptions on the use of the Health Guardian for Longevity Program to sustain health in West Africa. *COJ Nursing & Healthcare, 7*(3). https://doi.org/10.31031/COJNH.2021.07.000665

Chapter 4

Knowledge Management, Quality Improvement, and Technology Advancements

A Comprehensive Exploration

Introduction

The purpose of Chapter 4 is to deepen our understanding of health care informatics by exploring critical topics that bridge the gap between theory and practice. This chapter aims to equip us with practical knowledge and tools to navigate and excel in the ever-evolving field of HCIS, focusing on the current state and future direction of these systems, computer systems, and data management to enhance our ability to implement effective strategies for organizational success in the health care domain.

The significance of Chapter 4 lies in its comprehensive approach to crucial areas of health care informatics. It builds on the historical context, constructivist principles, and strategic planning insights gathered in previous chapters, providing a holistic view that connects foundational theories to real-world applications. This chapter empowers us to drive change and innovation, ultimately improving health care delivery and outcomes through enhanced knowledge management, quality improvement (QI), strategic planning, and workflow optimization.

Chapter 4 takes our understanding to new heights by building on the foundation established in the previous chapters. We've explored the history of computer technology's impact on health care and gained a contextual understanding of the field's evolution in Chapter 1. In Chapter 2, we delved into the constructivist principles of learning HCIS. We comprehensively covered topics such as computer systems, interoperability, integration, database management, structured and unstructured data, configuration, information management, health-related programs, data sources, elements, schemas, and analysis. Recognizing the significance of these components, we acknowledged how vital they are in achieving the desired outcomes, including creating mobile technology, enhancing access to quality health care, promoting sustainability, empowering patients, and enabling advanced fiscal and project management in diverse health venues. Chapter 3 shifted the spotlight to strategic and tactical planning, equipping you with essential knowledge and skills for effectively using digital tools within health-related programs. We emphasized the significance of planning for the successful implementation and utilization of HIS and HIT.

And now, in Chapter 4, we embark on an exploration of vital topics in health care informatics. Building on our previous discussions, our journey begins with understanding knowledge management and its transformative impact on organizations. We'll delve into strategies, tools, and technologies that enable effective knowledge management, drawing insights from real-world case scenarios. Next, we focus on QI, exploring frameworks like Six Sigma and Lean to understand their significance in health care settings. Through practical examples, we uncover tools and techniques for successful QI projects.

Building on this foundation, we recap the purpose and components of the logic model, a potent tool for program planning and evaluation. Practical applications and case scenarios provide insights into implementation. We also emphasize work plans in project management and their importance, key elements, and the ability to develop, monitor, and adapt them using real-life examples.

We then turn to the Technology Informatics Guiding Education Reform (TIGER) initiative, a force driving health care informatics. We discuss goals, objectives, impact, successes, challenges, and future directions shaped by TIGER.

Finally, we explore workflow optimization's significance in informatics. Insights into key concepts, analysis, mapping techniques, and the role of technology help streamline processes. Real-world examples illuminate successful workflow improvement initiatives. This comprehensive exploration empowers us to drive change and innovation in health care informatics effectively.

Objectives That Lead to Outcomes

By clearly distinguishing between process-oriented objectives and result-oriented outcomes, it becomes easier to understand and measure both the actions taken and the results achieved. Thus, the following table aligns key objectives with their corresponding outcomes, providing a clear and detailed understanding of what learners should achieve and comprehend upon completion. This alignment ensures that each objective is met with a tangible and measurable outcome, enhancing the overall learning experience.

Objective	Outcome
Define the concept of knowledge management and explain its importance in organizational success.	Understand the significance of knowledge management for achieving organizational success.
Identify strategies and techniques for effectively managing knowledge within an organization.	Develop and implement effective knowledge management strategies.
Evaluate the benefits and challenges of implementing knowledge management initiatives.	Assess the pros and cons of knowledge management initiatives in organizational contexts.
Understand the concept of QI and its significance in enhancing organizational performance.	Recognize the importance of QI for organizational performance enhancement.
Examine different QI frameworks and models, such as Six Sigma and Lean, and their applications.	Apply various QI models to organizational processes.

Define the purpose and components of a logic model.	Understand and articulate the purpose and components of a logic model for program evaluation.
Develop a comprehensive work plan by setting clear goals, defining specific tasks, and establishing timelines and allocating necessary resources.	Produce effective work plans that enhance project execution and contribute to overall organizational success.
Gain an overview of the TIGER initiative and its objectives in advancing health care informatics.	Understand the objectives of the TIGER initiative and its impact on health care informatics.

Key Terms

Directions: Before reading, please look at this list of key terms that will be used in this chapter. If any term is unfamiliar, please see the glossary at the end of the book.

knowledge management
logic model
quality improvement (QI)
TIGER
workflow
work plan

Historical Perspective of Knowledge Management

As we journey through the captivating history of knowledge management, we trace its origins to the early 20th century. Initially focused on managing organized information, the late 1980s and 1990s marked its emergence as a distinct field. Visionaries like Peter Drucker and the socialization, externalization, combination, internalization (SECI) model proponents enlightened us about leveraging explicit and tacit knowledge for a competitive edge (Farnese et al., 2019).

The late 1990s and early 2000s brought a shift and began treating knowledge as a strategic asset. The rise of the internet and digital technologies further accelerated sharing and disseminating knowledge, transforming economies into knowledge-based ones. Health care providers now recognize the importance of staying current with research and technology, equipping them to offer cutting-edge medical solutions.

This transition catalyzed technology integration into health care. From telemedicine facilitating remote consultations to AI-powered diagnostic tools, evolution hinges on research, technology, and human expertise synergy. Health care's economic expansion results from data-driven collaborative research, interdisciplinary collaboration, and technological advancements.

This shift's influence on health care is profound. The fusion of knowledge, technology, and expertise redefines health care's value proposition, enabling adaptation and innovation in a competitive landscape. Health care leverages technology to enhance patient care, driving advancements intertwined with evolving knowledge and information. In essence, the internet and digital technologies' impact led to a fundamental shift, making knowledge a central driver of economic success and emphasizing education, research, development, and technology's effective use.

Knowledge management seamlessly integrated itself into organizational practices, spanning human resources, training, and innovation management. Cultivating cultures that prioritize knowledge sharing and nurturing communities of practice emerged as vital strategies, fostering collaborative learning and expertise exchange (Schutt, 2003). The emergence of Web 2.0 technologies and social media marked a participatory shift, giving rise to social knowledge management. This approach nurtured collaboration, sharing, and collective wisdom.

Advancing alongside technology, knowledge management embraced new dimensions. AI, ML, and data analytics became integral, enhancing knowledge discovery and utilization capabilities. Scholars like Donald Berwick, renowned for his 1983 contributions to QI in health care, championed the continuous evolution of knowledge management and QI (Creighton, 2023). This brings us to the present, when knowledge management thrives and adapts to dynamic business landscapes. Agility and adaptability are paramount as we navigate intricate knowledge management across platforms, remote teams, and global contexts. Now that you have this historical perspective, you are better prepared to grasp the significance of knowledge management in our field of informatics. Let us carry this knowledge with us as we venture into the exciting world of managing and harnessing information for the betterment of our digital society!

In nursing informatics, the data, information, knowledge, and wisdom (DIKW) model, as proposed by Barclay and Murray in 1997, provides a small yet insightful window into how we navigate the complexities of knowledge management. By comprehending the progression illustrated from initial data transformation into information, then knowledge, and finally to the ultimate stage of wisdom, we attain a valuable perspective on enhancing communication and facilitating effective decision-making. This, in turn, results in improved outcomes.

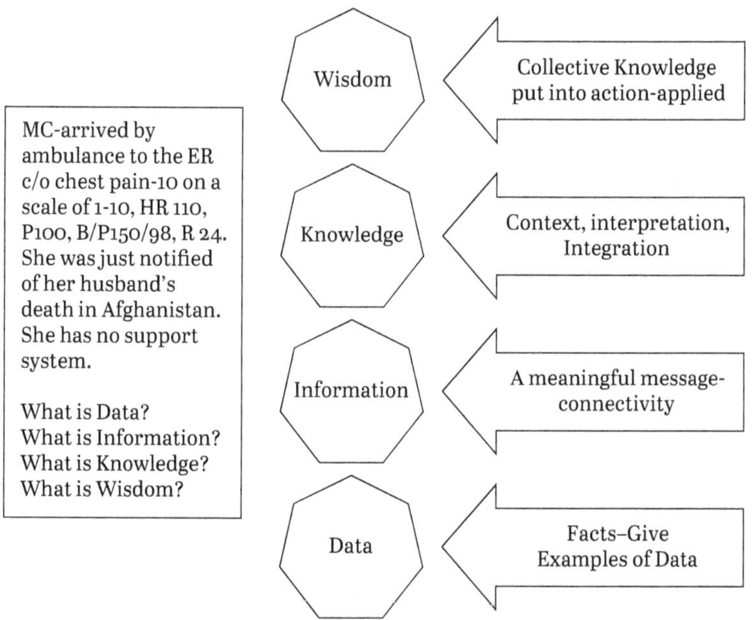

FIGURE 4.1 The DIKW model in practice.

Knowledge Management

In the realm of health care informatics, knowledge management emerges as a pivotal concept. Its essence lies in capturing, organizing, and sharing knowledge within health care organizations. This process is akin to arranging your study notes for easy access—a tangible analogy to illustrate the practice. Imagine you're a health care professional entrusted with critical decisions affecting patient outcomes. Equipped with the right knowledge, you possess a superpower! Knowledge management ensures access to the latest pertinent information for you and your peers—best practices, research findings, patient data—amplifying informed and effective decision-making.

However, the scope extends beyond individual knowledge. Collaboration proves indispensable in health care, especially within multidisciplinary teams delivering top-tier care. Knowledge management fosters teamwork by establishing systems enabling expertise exchange, breaking down departmental barriers, and enhancing overall efficiency.

Knowledge management possesses an intriguing facet—its power to stimulate innovation. When health care organizations systematically organize and analyze extensive knowledge, they unearth emerging trends and practices akin to discovering hidden treasures (Nonaka,1994). This invaluable insight spurs the genesis of novel ideas and solutions, pushing health care informatics' boundaries and propelling the field forward with innovative strides. This practice empowers health care organizations to reflect, discern effective strategies, and learn from failures—akin to personal growth through acknowledging mistakes.

In essence, the goal remains elevating patient care quality and crafting successful programs within health care informatics' captivating realm. Your journey of learning and exploration can profoundly impact the health care arena. Managing knowledge within an organization is pivotal for success, and numerous strategies facilitate this endeavor. Let's delve into some of the most effective ones.

EFFECTIVE KNOWLEDGE MANAGEMENT STRATEGIES AND TECHNIQUES

- *Knowledge-sharing platforms*: Creating platforms like intranet sites or online forums on which employees can share their knowledge, experiences, and ideas with each other. It's like having a virtual meeting space where everyone can contribute their valuable insights.
- *Communities of practice*: Encouraging the formation of communities within the organization where people with similar interests or expertise can collaborate and exchange knowledge. These communities act like support groups where members can learn from each other.
- *Knowledge mapping*: Identifying and documenting the knowledge that exists within the organization, like a treasure map that helps everyone know what valuable information is available and where to find it.
- *Learning and training programs*: Offering regular learning sessions and training opportunities for employees to acquire new knowledge and skills—just like attending classes to boost your expertise!
- *Mentorship and coaching*: Pairing experienced employees with newer ones so that knowledge and expertise can be transferred from one generation to the next, like a seasoned traveler guiding a novice.
- *Knowledge capture*: Creating mechanisms to capture knowledge from experts before they retire or move to other positions. It's like preserving the wisdom of the elders for future generations.
- *Knowledge champions*: Appointing individuals who are passionate about knowledge management to take the lead and promote its importance within the organization. They act as cheerleaders, spreading the enthusiasm for knowledge management.
- *Recognition and rewards*: Acknowledging and rewarding employees who actively share their knowledge and contribute to the organization's

learning culture. It's like giving a high-five to those who go the extra mile!

- *Collaborative projects*: Encouraging cross-functional or interdisciplinary projects so that employees from different areas work together. This fosters knowledge exchange and brings fresh perspectives.
- *After-action reviews*: After completing projects or tasks, holding discussions to analyze what worked well and what could be improved. It's like a postgame analysis to learn from both successes and challenges.

Knowledge management fosters a culture of learning and sharing, transforming organizations into thriving hubs of knowledge, leading to continuous growth and success. Collaboration and knowledge sharing unlock an organization's full potential, driving innovation and improvement across processes.

Understanding QI and Its Impact on Organizational Performance

QI

As our exploration continues, knowledge management seamlessly converges with QI—an equally vital concept for organizations aspiring to excel. QI centers on achieving heightened efficiency and effectiveness. Like knowledge management, it involves identifying areas for enhancement and executing targeted actions for superior outcomes.

Imagine a scenario: In your journey as future informatics professionals, you engage in projects for which you've developed cutting-edge health care software aiming to enhance patient care and streamline medical processes. Despite earnest efforts, post–initial implementation, feedback surfaces from health care professionals and users. Usability issues, system crashes, and functionality concerns emerge. While beneficial in numerous aspects, these glitches hinder medical staff from effective use, impacting overall patient care quality. QI intersects with health care technology.

QI, in this context, entails pinpointing challenges faced by health care professionals, patients, and the health care system as a whole. It mandates specific actions to address these challenges and bolster application performance. Seeking input from users—doctors, nurses, administrators—yields valuable insights into strengths and weaknesses. Analyzing this feedback identifies root causes and prioritizes areas for enhancement.

Collaboration with health care professionals and technology experts aids in innovative solutions. Iterative processes mend bugs, streamline workflows, and augment features for enhanced user-friendliness, reliability, and efficiency. Regular updates in health care tech applications are essential for optimal patient care and medical support.

By observing your team's QI initiatives, the application evolves, aligning with diverse health care settings' distinct requirements. The outcome? Improved patient outcomes, elevated efficiency, and a culture of continuous learning within the organization.

Integrating QI into health care tech development is pivotal. Committing to enhancing application quality yields a tangible impact on patient care, fostering advancements in health care technology. So, why is QI significant? Here are several reasons:

EVALUATE BENEFITS OF QI

- *Customer satisfaction*: When organizations improve the quality of their products or services, it leads to greater customer satisfaction. Satisfied customers are more likely to return and recommend the organization to others, which helps build a loyal customer base.
- *Efficiency and productivity*: QI often involves streamlining processes and eliminating waste. By doing so, organizations become more productive, using their resources effectively to achieve better results.

- *Cost reduction*: When organizations identify and fix problems, they can reduce the costs associated with errors, defects, and rework. This can lead to cost savings and more resources available for further improvements.
- *Competitive advantage*: Organizations that focus on QI gain a competitive edge in the market. When they consistently deliver better products or services, they stand out from their competitors, attracting more customers and achieving long-term success.
- *Employee morale*: QI efforts involve employees at all levels of the organization. When employees see that their input and efforts lead to positive changes and better outcomes, it boosts their morale and engagement.
- *Organizational reputation*: A track record of delivering high-quality products or services enhances an organization's reputation. A positive reputation attracts more customers and partners, creating new opportunities for growth.

QI is a crucial aspect of any successful organization and a staple in most practices that lead to successful outcomes. It helps us meet customer expectations, operate efficiently, reduce costs, and stay ahead of the competition. By continually striving to improve, organizations can enhance their performance and achieve long-term success.

In the realm of health care, the pursuit of excellence in patient care and operational efficiency is at the core of success. QI methodologies play a pivotal role in achieving these goals, and when combined with health informatics, the impact becomes even more profound.

Through health informatics, we harness the power of technology and data to revolutionize health care delivery. By integrating informatics into our practices, we can make well-informed decisions, optimize processes, and transform the patient experience.

Now let's explore two influential frameworks that align perfectly with health informatics: Six Sigma and Lean. Six Sigma is a data-driven approach that meticulously analyzes health data to identify and eliminate defects and variations in processes. By using statistical tools and the define, measure, analyze, improve, and control (DMAIC) methodology, we can diagnose issues with precision and improve patient outcomes. From reducing medication errors to enhancing diagnostic accuracy, Six Sigma empowers us to raise the bar of care.

In contrast, Lean methodology complements Six Sigma's analytical prowess by focusing on waste elimination and process optimization. In health care, Lean principles work hand in hand with health informatics to minimize waiting times, allocate resources efficiently, and create a seamless patient journey. Through value stream mapping and just-in-time production, we ensure patients receive the right care at the right time.

Different QI Framework and Models

As aspiring health care professionals, grasping the symbiotic relationship between health informatics and QI is crucial. Nurturing a culture of perpetual enhancement empowers us to remain at the vanguard of medical progress and provide exemplary, patient-centered care. The fusion of health informatics and QI positively shapes the future of health care. By embracing the transformative principles of Six Sigma and Lean, we embark on a journey to enhance patient care, reduce costs, and make a lasting impact in the lives of those we serve. Let us wholeheartedly embrace these principles as we prepare to be change-makers in tomorrow's health care arena.

While delving into QI frameworks like Six Sigma and Lean, their striking resemblances to scientific problem solving, research, and algorithms become evident. Imagine this moment as a luminous "Eureka!" within the realm of health informatics—a realization that the principles you're absorbing are intricately intertwined with the essence of scientific investigation and analysis. Just as scientists keenly observe and analyze data to uncover insights and solve mysteries of the natural world, Six Sigma employs a data-driven approach to meticulously scrutinize health care data. By applying statistical tools and the DMAIC cycle, we dissect complex health care processes to identify and eliminate defects, similar to a scientist pinpointing the root cause of a scientific puzzle.

Your journey in health informatics has illuminated the significance of research methodologies and optimizing processes for more efficient outcomes. Interestingly, Lean methodology echoes this pursuit of efficiency by emphasizing waste elimination and streamlined health care practices. Just as researchers refine their methodologies, Lean empowers health care professionals to do the same, ensuring timely and effective patient care. Remarkably, the algorithms guiding you through precise informatics steps unveil a parallel with Six Sigma's DMAIC cycle. While algorithms lead to solutions, DMAIC guides us on a data-driven journey toward process improvement, ultimately enhancing patient outcomes and operational efficiency. This pursuit of excellence is a foundation of QI, as continuous enhancement of health care practices remains a constant goal.

As you connect the dots and witness the convergence of scientific problem solving, research, and algorithms with health informatics and QI, let this "Aha!" moment inspire you. Embrace the synergy of these disciplines, for within it lies the key to becoming truly exceptional health care professionals.

This profound connection underscores health informatics' transformative potential in shaping health care's future. Allow this revelation to guide you, illuminating the path toward innovation, optimization, and delivering the highest quality of patient-centered care. With this newfound awareness, you're poised to catalyze change, steering the health care industry toward a future when technology, data, and compassion intersect, fostering healthier and happier lives.

As students exploring health informatics and QI, recognize that enhancing health application quality profoundly impacts patient care outcomes. By incorporating QI principles, you have the opportunity to make a real difference in health care technology advancement.

Now let's delve into a compelling scenario showcasing successful QI efforts in health informatics. This scenario centers on a 400-bed urban hospital grappling with patient care quality challenges.

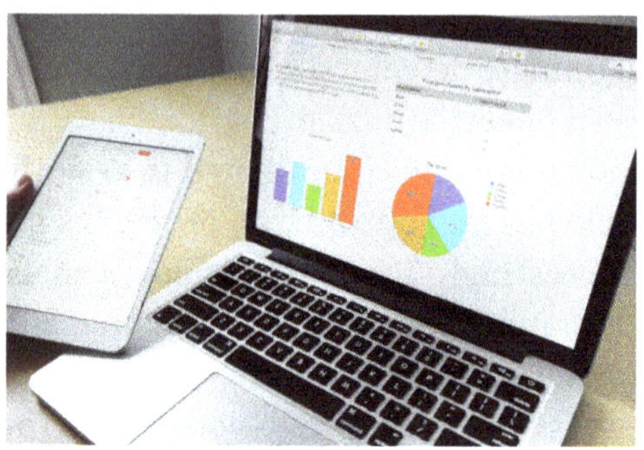

FIGURE 4.2 Metrics and measurements.

Recognizing health informatics' potential, the hospital implements an encompassing system, including an EHR system, computerized physician order entry (CPOE), and clinical decision support systems (CDSS). Through this scenario, you'll gain insights into measurement and metrics' pivotal role in assessing and monitoring QI initiatives, ultimately transforming patient care outcomes and advancing health informatics.

Measurement and Metrics Implementation

Before implementing the HIS, understanding measurement and metrics implementation in health informatics is vital. This knowledge is crucial for your role as future informatics professionals to enhance patient care and hospital efficiency. As you enter the realm of health informatics, recognizing the importance of baseline data collection is essential. The hospital's QI team collects data on KPIs before implementing the HIS. These KPIs include readmission rates, medication errors, patient satisfaction scores, and average length of stay. This baseline helps evaluate the informatics initiatives' impact effectively.

As informatics professionals, identifying key metrics during and after implementation becomes pivotal. These metrics are crucial for monitoring and evaluating the informatics system's success. Key metrics include EHR adoption rates, CPOE usage frequency, CDSS alert response rates, and system uptime. Monitoring these metrics allows proactive problem solving.

Once the health informatics system is operational, real-time monitoring becomes integral. Interactive dashboards track the system's performance across departments and among individuals. Regularly reviewing these dashboards detects issues promptly.

Collaborating with health care professionals and gathering feedback is paramount. Staff feedback is invaluable. Surveys and feedback provide insights into system usability and effectiveness, guiding improvements to meet health care professionals' needs.

Analyzing collected data reveals health informatics' impact on patient care quality. Standardized processes and CDSS automated alerts enhance patient outcomes and reduce readmission rates. Health informatics streamlines clinical workflows, decreasing the average length of stay and increasing patient throughput.

While implementing health informatics, challenges may arise, such as initial resistance from health care professionals. Proper training and support are vital for successful adoption.

Continuous improvement is also integral to health informatics. Based on feedback and data, identifying areas for enhancement and collaborating with your team optimizes the system's functionality. As future informatics professionals, cost-effectiveness plays a role in your decision-making. Although initial investment exists, health informatics proves cost-effective over time due to improved patient care and reduced medical errors.

Measurement and metrics implementation holds a central role in your future as graduate informatics students. This knowledge equips you to assess and monitor QI through health informatics. Embrace learning and growth, as your contributions in health informatics can enhance patient care and transform health care delivery.

Now let's delve into practical application by creating a logic model for a 400-bed urban hospital implementing a comprehensive health informatics system. Understanding logical patterns and key metrics prepares you to drive improvements in patient care and hospital efficiency.

As the health informatics initiative progresses, the hospital administration closely monitors data collected from the new HIT systems.

TABLE 4.1 Logic Model: Enhancing Patient Care Quality Through Health Informatics

Inputs	Activities	Outputs	Outcomes	Impact
• Skilled health informatics team • Adequate funding for health informatics implementation • Advanced HIT systems: ◦ EHR system ◦ CPOE ◦ CDSS ◦ Hospital data and resources	• Assess the hospital's existing workflow and identify areas for improvement • Customize and integrate the EHR, CPOE, and CDSS systems into the hospital's operations • Conduct extensive training for hospital staff to ensure effective utilization of the new HIT system • Implement data collection mechanisms and protocols for patient information capture • Collaborate with health care professionals to ensure the seamless adoption of new systems	• Successful customization and integration of EHR, CPOE, and CDSS into hospital workflows • Well-trained hospital staff proficient in using the HIT systems • Comprehensive patient data collected and accessible through the EHR system • Enhanced collaboration among health care professionals through HIT-enabled communication	• Short-term: Streamlined data entry and retrieval processes, reducing administrative burden • Intermediate: Increased accuracy and accessibility of patient data, leading to improved care coordination • Long-term: Reduced medical errors and enhanced patient safety through clinical decision support	• Improved patient care quality and safety • Enhanced efficiency in hospital operations • Increased patient satisfaction and positive feedback • Enhanced reputation and trust in the hospital's services

This includes metrics related to patient outcomes, medical errors, staff satisfaction, and financial efficiency. The logic model reveals the program's theory of change, enabling stakeholders to understand objectives and expected outcomes. It fosters accountability among the health informatics team and hospital management, tracking progress and ensuring success. The logic model guides continuous improvement. Data analysis identifies areas for optimization and refinement of HIT systems, aligning with evolving health care system needs and goals. Using logic models in QI ensures systematic evaluation of health informatics interventions, driving sustainable improvements in patient care and hospital performance.

Understanding the significance of work plans in project management and organizational success is crucial. Work plans act as navigational charts, guiding project execution like blueprints to achieve goals effectively and efficiently. In project management, work plans detail elements that shape the endeavor's course. From clear, measurable goals and objectives to defining tasks, the work plan structures the program. Creating work plans starts with defining goals and objectives with clarity.

TABLE 4.2 Standard Work Plan

Section	Details
Goal:	
Measurable Outcome(s):	
Time Frame:	
Major Objectives, Key Tasks:	
Person Responsible (Including Deadlines Given)	

Note: Setting SMART goals keeps efforts focused. Allocating tasks according to team strengths helps maintain a shared vision. Work plans establish timelines and allocate resources, tracking progress. Regular monitoring detects deviations, allowing for adaptations to changes. Flexibility is key for handling unexpected challenges.

Work Plans and Logic Models

Work plans guide the journey, while logic models provide a panoramic view of inputs, activities, outputs, outcomes, and impact. Together, elements of knowledge management, QI, logic models, work plans, and workflow form a holistic approach to advancing health care practices and patient outcomes. An initiative exemplifying this interconnectedness is the TIGER.

Adapting Practices for Better Health Care

TIGER aims to enhance the integration of technology and knowledge management into nursing practice, transforming patient care and clinical decision-making (Hübner et al., 2018). TIGER's impact on nursing practice and health care delivery is significant. By promoting technology and evidence-based practices, it empowers nurses to provide patient-centered care and interdisciplinary collaboration. Though successful, TIGER faces implementation challenges due to the complexity of integration and training needs. These challenges provide learning opportunities for more effective strategies.

Understanding Interconnectedness and the TIGER Initiative

TIGER shapes health care informatics with trends like telehealth and advances in technology. Professionals must adapt practices for better health care delivery, with far-reaching implications.

The TIGER initiative is a beacon of innovation for a future when health care informatics empowers professionals and enhances patient outcomes. Comprehending its objectives equips us for a digitally driven health care landscape. As we embrace this journey, let's unlock the potential of informatics, addressing health care challenges and serving underserved communities.

Summary

Chapter 4 elucidates the interconnectedness of health care informatics, knowledge management, QI, logic models, work plans, and the TIGER initiative, offering insights and strategies that equip health care professionals to navigate the dynamic landscape of modern health care. By integrating these elements, professionals can enhance decision-making, streamline workflows, and drive meaningful improvements in patient care and system efficiency.

Chapter Review Questions

Directions: Consider what you learned in this chapter as you respond to the health care scenario and questions.

Health Care Scenario: EHR System Project for Small Clinics

Imagine you are a project manager for a mid-sized health care IT company. Your team has been tasked with creating a new EHR system designed to improve workflow and efficiency for small clinics. The project is slated to take 6 months, and you are currently at the end of the 2nd month. The project has four main phases: planning, development, testing, and deployment.

Your team has completed the planning phase and is midway through the development phase. During a routine status meeting, the following issues were raised:

> **Issue 1:** One of the senior developers, who has extensive experience with health care regulations, has unexpectedly left the company, causing a potential delay in the development timeline.
>
> **Issue 2:** A new, more secure coding framework has been released that could significantly improve the project, but it would require redoing some of the work already completed.
>
> **Issue 3:** A key stakeholder, a leading clinic, has requested an additional feature that was not part of the original project scope.

Given these issues, you need to make informed decisions to keep the project on track and ensure its successful completion.

Multiple-Choice Questions

1. Considering issue 1, how should you address the senior developer's departure to minimize delays?

    a. Reassign tasks to the remaining team members and work overtime.
    b. Hire a freelance developer with health care experience temporarily.
    c. Negotiate a project timeline extension with stakeholders.
    d. Focus on the tasks that can be completed without the senior developer.

2. In light of issue 2, what is the best course of action regarding the new secure coding framework?

    a. Ignore the new framework and continue with the current plan.
    b. Switch to the new framework immediately, redoing the necessary work.
    c. Conduct a cost-benefit analysis to determine the impact of switching.
    d. Postpone the decision until the next project.

3. How should you handle the key stakeholder's request for an additional feature (issue 3)?

    a. Add the feature without adjusting the project scope or timeline.
    b. Refuse the request to keep the project on track.
    c. Assess the impact on the project scope, timeline, and resources, and discuss with the stakeholder.
    d. Delegate the request to another team to handle separately.

4. Given the departure of the senior developer, what is a key consideration when reassessing the project timeline and tasks?

    a. Focusing solely on completing the project as quickly as possible

b. Ensuring all team members are equally busy
c. Balancing the quality of the final product with the project deadlines
d. Avoiding any changes to the initial project plan

5. How can you ensure that the project remains aligned with its goals despite the challenges?

    a. Frequently changing the project plan to accommodate new challenges
    b. Sticking rigidly to the original plan regardless of obstacles
    c. Regularly reviewing and adjusting the project plan while keeping the goals in focus
    d. Delegating decision-making to individual team members to increase efficiency

6. What steps can you take to manage the impact of the senior developer's departure on team morale?

    a. Ignore the issue and continue as planned.
    b. Hold a team meeting to discuss the situation and gather input on solutions.
    c. Assign additional work to the remaining team members without acknowledgment.
    d. Replace the senior developer immediately without involving the team.

7. How should you prioritize tasks in light of the request for an additional feature?

    a. Complete the requested feature first, regardless of the impact on other tasks.
    b. Prioritize tasks based on their importance to the overall project goals.
    c. Delay all other tasks until the additional feature is completed.
    d. Equally divide time between all tasks without consideration of importance.

Answer Key

1. (b) Hire a freelance developer with health care experience temporarily.
2. (c) Conduct a cost-benefit analysis to determine the impact of switching.
3. (c) Assess the impact on the project scope, timeline, and resources, and discuss with the stakeholder.
4. (c) Balancing the quality of the final product with the project deadlines
5. (c) Regularly reviewing and adjusting the project plan while keeping the goals in focus
6. (b) Hold a team meeting to discuss the situation and gather input on solutions.
7. (b) Prioritize tasks based on their importance to the overall project goals.

References

Barclay, R. O., & Murray, P. C. (1997). *What is knowledge management?* http://www.providersedge.com/docs/km_articles/what_is_knowledge_management.pdf

Creighton, S. (2023). Don Berwick: Founder of the Institute for Health care Improvement (IHI). *LifeQI*. https://blog.lifeqisystem.com/don-berwick

Farnese, M. L., Barbieri, B., Chirumbolo, A., & Patriotta, G. (2019). Managing knowledge in organizations: A Nonaka's SECI model operationalization. *Frontiers in Psychology, 10*, 2730. https://doi.org/10.3389/fpsyg.2019.02730

Hübner, U., Shaw, T., Thye, J., Egbert, N., Marin, H. F., Chang, P., O'Connor, S., Day, K., Honey, M., Blake, R., Hovenga, E., Skiba, D., & Ball, M. J. (2018). Technology informatics guiding education reform - TIGER. *Methods of Information in Medicine, 57*(1), e30–e42. https://doi.org/10.3414/ME17-01-0155

Nonaka, I. (1994). A dynamic theory of organizational knowledge creation. *Organization Science, 5*(1), 14–37.

Schutt, P. (2003). The post-nonAka knowledge management. *Journal of Universal Computer Science, 9*(6), 1–12.

Figure Credit

Fig. 4.2: Copyright © 2016 Pexels/Pixabay.

Chapter 5

Navigating the HIS Life Cycle and Project Management Principles

Introduction

The purpose of Chapter 5 is to bridge the gap between theoretical knowledge and the practical implementation of HIS projects. This chapter aims to provide a detailed understanding of the precise steps and strategic decisions necessary for executing HIS projects successfully. It also emphasizes the importance of maintaining ongoing product development and support postlaunch, a critical yet often overlooked aspect. By exploring concepts such as strategy, tactics, project management, system selection, project scoping, fast-track methods, implementation, maintenance, development oversight, and decision-making for changes, this chapter equips students with the skills and knowledge needed for effective HIS project management within the ever-evolving health care landscape.

Chapter 5 is significant because it delves into the practical aspects of managing and implementing HIS projects, providing students with the tools to navigate the complexities of these systems effectively. This chapter highlights the importance of strategic and tactical planning, project management, and organizational skills in ensuring the success of HIS projects. It underscores the necessity of assembling the right team, defining project scope, detailing project plans, and employing fast-track methods to accelerate development and deployment. Additionally, it addresses the crucial role of ongoing maintenance and development, as well as the decision-making processes that lead to changes in HIS products. By offering case scenarios and practical insights, Chapter 5 prepares students to contribute actively to the successful realization and evolution of HIS within the dynamic health care environment, ultimately enhancing processes, patient care, and the overall health care landscape.

As we continue our exploration of HIS in this fifth chapter, we build on the foundational knowledge you've acquired in previous chapters. In Chapters 1–4, we uncovered the significance of HIS in modern health care, delved into the complexities of strategic and tactical information planning, and became familiar with the pivotal role of a systematic system selection task force. We also witnessed the collaborative efforts involved in defining the scope of a HIS project and finalizing its intricate details. Additionally, we explored innovative fast-track design-and-build methods that expedite project realization while maintaining a focus on quality and precision.

Chapter 5 serves as your gateway to understanding the system life cycle of a HIS and the principles of project management and organization. The system life cycle encompasses stages ranging from planning and design to implementation, maintenance, and retirement. These stages involve identifying needs and goals, creating comprehensive designs, installing and configuring systems, rigorous testing, ongoing support, and eventual decommissioning, if necessary.

The principles of project management and organization encompass techniques for planning, executing, and controlling projects. These principles involve setting clear goals and objectives, developing a project plan, establishing a budget, and managing resources and risks.

By studying the system life cycle of HIS and understanding the principles of project management and organization, you will gain valuable insights into how to effectively develop and manage these critical systems. This knowledge will empower you to navigate the world of HIS with greater clarity, ensuring a smoother journey for both you and the patients who rely on these systems for their health care needs.

Objectives That Lead to Outcomes

We have outlined specific objectives and their corresponding expected outcomes for this chapter. The following table aligns key objectives with their outcomes, providing a clear and detailed understanding of what learners should achieve and comprehend upon completion. This alignment ensures that each objective is met with a tangible and measurable outcome, enhancing the overall learning experience. These objectives will guide the planning and execution of the HIS project, ensuring it aligns with the organization's strategic goals and principles of effective project management and organizational management.

Objective	Outcome
Develop a comprehensive strategic information plan that aligns the HIS with the organization's long-term goals, focusing on data management, technology infrastructure, and resource allocation.	A well-defined strategic plan that aligns with long-term goals, ensuring efficient data management, robust technology infrastructure, and optimal resource allocation.
Create a tactical information plan outlining short- to medium-term strategies for HIS implementation, including software and hardware upgrades, staff training, and data security measures.	An actionable tactical plan that addresses immediate needs such as software and hardware upgrades, staff training, and enhanced data security.
Understand and apply key principles of project and organization management to ensure the successful implementation and maintenance of the HIS, emphasizing resource allocation, risk management, and stakeholder communication.	Effective project and organizational management leading to successful HIS implementation, with well-managed resources, minimized risks, and clear stakeholder communication.
Establish a cross-functional task force responsible for evaluating, selecting, and recommending the most suitable HIS system based on the organization's specific needs, budget constraints, and technical requirements.	A dedicated task force providing well-researched recommendations for the most suitable HIS system, ensuring it meets specific needs and budget constraints.

Reach a consensus among stakeholders regarding the scope, objectives, and deliverables of the HIS project, ensuring clarity and alignment with organizational goals.	Unified stakeholder agreement on the HIS project scope, objectives, and deliverables, ensuring clarity and alignment with organizational goals.
Define project details such as timelines, budgets, roles, responsibilities, and performance metrics to ensure effective project planning and execution.	Detailed project plan with clear timelines, budgets, roles, responsibilities, and performance metrics, facilitating efficient project execution.

Key Terms

Directions: Before reading, please look at this list of key terms that will be used in this chapter. If any term is unfamiliar, please see the glossary at the end of the book.

agreement on the scope of the project
change decision
development
fast-track methods
finalization of project details
implementation
maintenance
management
project details
project management
project scope
strategy
system selection team
tactics

Introduction to Systems' Life Cycles

Now that we've laid the groundwork for understanding HIS and the principles of project management and organization, it's time to delve into a crucial aspect of HIS implementation—the system life cycle. In previous chapters, you gained insights into HIS significance, strategic planning, tactical information planning, and the essentials of project management. You also learned about the system selection team, project scope, project details, fast-track methods, implementation, maintenance, development, and change decisions—key components of effective HIS project management (Wager et al., 2022).

Before diving into the life cycle of these systems, it's important to distinguish HIS from HCIS. HIS serves as an overarching framework for collecting, managing, and analyzing health-related data at various levels, including public health databases and research platforms. HCIS, on the other hand, is a subset of HIS, specifically designed to support clinical and administrative functions within health care organizations, such as EHRs and patient management systems. Understanding this distinction is essential for navigating system development and implementation.

In this chapter, we'll take a deep dive into the HIS life cycle. These stages are the building blocks of successful HCIS, encompassing strategic planning, system design, project execution, and continuous support. Throughout this chapter, you'll not only grasp the theoretical aspects of the HIS life cycle, but also gain practical insights into how these principles apply in real-world HIS projects. This knowledge will equip you to confidently navigate the complexities of HIS implementation, ensuring that these critical systems effectively serve their roles in the ever-evolving health care landscape.

You will further enhance your understanding of key components such as the system selection team, project scope, project details, fast-track methods, implementation, maintenance, development, and change decisions within the realm of effective HIS project management.

The HIS Life Cycle Process

First and foremost, you'll create a detailed project description. Think of this as crafting a roadmap that clearly defines what your project aims to achieve. This description serves as a beacon, guiding your team toward the desired destination.

Then, you'll delve into specifying project deliverables and outcomes. By outlining precisely what will be produced during the project, you set expectations and milestones. This step ensures that everyone knows what success looks like.

To prevent any misunderstandings or scope creep, you'll define scope boundaries. This process distinguishes what's included within the project and what falls outside its purview. This clarity is essential for keeping the project on track.

Roles and responsibilities come next. Here, you'll clarify who does what during the project. This ensures that everyone knows their tasks and responsibilities, promoting efficiency and accountability within the team.

Lastly, you'll develop change-control processes. Projects often evolve, and it's vital to have a plan in place to manage changes to the project scope effectively. This proactive approach minimizes disruptions and keeps the project aligned with its objectives. With these steps, you'll not only set the project's course but also create a shared understanding among your team, setting the stage for a well-organized and successful HCIS project.

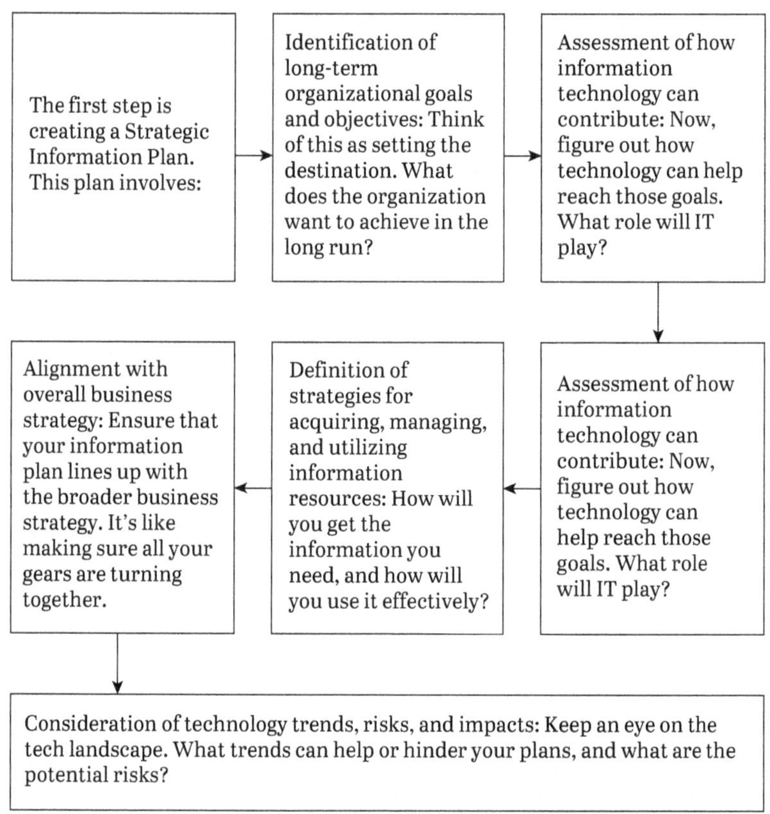

FIGURE 5.1 Following the pathway.

Tactical Information Plan

Now that we've laid the strategic foundation, let's shift our focus to the tactical information plan. This step involves detailed planning, technology selection, budgeting, scheduling, and ensuring effective team preparation—a practical blueprint that drives project success. In this phase, we move beyond theory and into action.

The tactical information plan comprises several key components that lay the groundwork for effective project execution. First, you will the importance of breaking down the big goals into specific, manageable steps and actions. These detailed plans and actions are the building blocks of your project's success, providing a clear roadmap for implementation. Next, you'll address the critical aspect of technology specifications. Choosing the right tools and systems for the job is crucial. You'll be guided through the process of making informed decisions to ensure that your chosen technology aligns with your project objectives. Budget allocation and resource planning also take center stage. Determining how much financial investment and human resources your initiatives require is a fundamental step in ensuring the project's viability.

The Timeline

To keep everything on track, a well-defined timeline for implementation is essential. You'll create a schedule with clear deadlines for each project element, ensuring that tasks are completed on time. Furthermore, you'll delve into the significance of user training, change management, and communication, preparing your team for the changes that come with project implementation and ensuring that everyone is aligned for success.

As you continue to explore the complexities of health care projects, you will shift your focus to the foundational principles of project management and organizational leadership. This step will introduce you to the core concepts, methodologies, and crucial skills required for effective project leadership and integration within a health care organization.

Within the realm of project management, you'll begin with a solid introduction to the basics of managing projects effectively. From there, you'll explore key project management principles, including scope, time, cost, quality, and more—these pillars support successful project execution.

You'll also gain insight into various project management methodologies, such as Agile and Waterfall, allowing you to adapt your approach to different project scenarios (Nelson & Staggers 2014). Understanding how project management integrates into an organization's structure is crucial for seamless implementation.

But it's not just about processes—leadership, communication, and risk management are equally essential skills for successful project management. This section will equip you with the knowledge and tools needed to lead and communicate effectively while mitigating risks.

As you navigate this journey through HCIS, one critical aspect stands out: selecting the right system. To achieve this, you'll assemble a system selection task force—experts with the necessary skills to guide the process. This team will play a central role in identifying the organization's true needs, establishing evaluation criteria, and comparing potential systems.

Your journey will involve a structured decision-making process, ensuring a clear and justified choice. Moreover, you'll finalize the project's scope, detailing objectives, specifying deliverables, defining boundaries, clarifying roles and responsibilities, planning for change control, and documenting everything comprehensively.

Additionally, you'll allocate resources effectively, assess risks, and maintain transparent communication throughout the project. These steps form the foundation for successful HCIS selection and implementation.

SYSTEM SELECTION TASK FORCE EXECUTION

When selecting the right system, you'll need the following:

- *Formation and composition of the task force*: Put together a team with the right expertise.
- *Identification of needs and requirements*: What does the organization truly need from the system?
- *Evaluation criteria*: Develop standards for assessing different system options.
- *Evaluation and comparison*: Assess the pros and cons of potential systems.
- *Decision-making process*: Make a clear, justified choice.

Now that we've explored the crucial role of forming a system selection task force and making informed choices, let's focus on ensuring everyone is on the same page regarding the scope of your HCIS project. This stage, often referred to as agreement on the scope of the project, lays the groundwork for a successful journey ahead.

AGREEMENT ON THE SCOPE OF THE PROJECT ESSENTIALS

- *Detailed project description*: Clearly define what the project aims to achieve.
- *Project deliverables and outcomes*: Specify what will be produced.
- *Scope boundaries*: Define what's included and what's not.
- *Roles and responsibilities*: Clarify who does what during the project.
- *Change-control processes*: Plan for managing changes to the project scope.

As we progress through the stages of developing a HCIS, the spotlight shifts to the finalization of project details. This phase is like putting the finishing touches on a complex puzzle, ensuring that every piece aligns perfectly for a successful outcome.

First and foremost, you'll focus on the refinement of plans. Think of this as meticulously fine-tuning your project's blueprint. It's crucial to ensure that all plans are not only detailed but also realistic. This step helps prevent unexpected roadblocks and keeps your project on track.

Next, you'll look at resource allocation—a critical aspect of project management. Here, you'll assign tasks and allocate resources to your team members based on their skills and capabilities. This process optimizes efficiency and ensures that each team member contributes effectively to the project's success. A comprehensive project plan document will be your guiding compass throughout this journey. Everything from goals to timelines, milestones, and responsibilities should be documented in detail. This written record provides clarity and accountability, making sure nothing gets overlooked.

Risk assessment comes next. In the dynamic world of HCIS, identifying potential problems and devising strategies to tackle them is essential. This proactive approach minimizes disruptions and ensures your project remains resilient in the face of challenges.

Lastly, you'll explore the development of a communication plan. Effective communication is the lifeblood of any project. You'll learn how to keep everyone informed, from team members to stakeholders, ensuring transparency, alignment, and a smooth flow of information throughout the project. By mastering these finalization steps, you'll not only fine-tune your project's execution, but also bolster your ability to navigate the complexities of HCIS development successfully.

FINALIZATION OF PROJECT DETAILS

- *Refinement of plans*: Make sure all plans are detailed and realistic.
- *Resource allocation*: Assign tasks and resources to your team members.
- *Comprehensive project plan document*: Put everything in writing.
- *Risk assessment*: Identify potential problems and how to deal with them.
- *Communication plan*: Keep everyone informed throughout the project.

Fast-Track Design-and-Build Methods in Health Care Informatics

In the realm of health care informatics, the ability to swiftly implement critical systems can significantly impact patient care, operational efficiency, and competitiveness in the rapidly evolving health care landscape. Fast-track project delivery methods prioritize speed and efficiency without compromising quality.

Consider a scenario when a health care organization urgently needs to upgrade its EHR system due to new regulatory requirements. Traditional project management typically follows a linear sequence: design, construct, and test. However, fast-track methods break this mold by allowing these phases to overlap. While design progresses, construction begins concurrently, significantly reducing project timelines.

This adaptability is a hallmark of fast-track methods. They embrace agility, recognizing that health care informatics projects often encounter changes due to new regulations, emerging technologies, or evolving patient needs. This allows teams to pivot swiftly and stay responsive in a dynamic environment.

The advantages of fast-tracking are compelling. It expedites project delivery, enabling health care organizations to implement critical systems sooner. This results in improved patient care, enhanced operational efficiency, and a competitive edge. Moreover, it can lead to cost savings by reducing project durations.

However, fast-track methods do come with their own set of challenges. Coordinating multiple teams concurrently requires meticulous planning and communication. There's also the risk of overlooking critical details during rapid phases. Effective management of potential disruptions arising from overlapping phases is crucial for project success.

Despite the need for speed, maintaining high-quality standards is non-negotiable in health care informatics. Fast-track projects must undergo rigorous quality assurance processes to ensure compliance with standards and regulatory requirements. Moreover, robust risk management strategies are vital. Fast-track projects demand proactive identification of potential risks early in the project's life cycle. Teams must assess risks' impact and develop mitigation plans to prevent setbacks and keep projects on course.

Fast-track project delivery methods offer an agile and efficient way to implement health care informatics projects swiftly. Understanding the principles, benefits, challenges, and risk management associated with fast-track methods equips students in health care informatics with the knowledge and skills needed for project management in this dynamic field.

Implementing the Project

Let's move into the implementation of the project. This is the moment when all the meticulous planning and preparation transform into action, propelling your health care informatics project forward.

First and foremost, you'll execute the tasks outlined in your project plan. It's like setting the gears in motion. This phase marks the commencement of the actual work, whether it's developing software, deploying hardware, or rolling out new health care processes.

As you move forward, you'll need to maintain a vigilant eye on progress. Monitoring becomes your constant companion, ensuring that the project is advancing as intended. Think of this as a navigational check to ensure you're staying on course.

Resource and budget management become paramount. Efficiently utilizing the allocated resources and staying within budget constraints is essential. This involves not only managing financial resources but also human resources and materials effectively.

In the dynamic landscape of health care informatics, issues and changes are almost inevitable. Therefore, issue management becomes a core task. When problems arise or unexpected changes occur, you need a structured approach to address them promptly and effectively.

Throughout this phase, your North Star remains the alignment with project objectives. It's vital to ensure that every action and decision is in harmony with the project's overarching goals. Regularly revisiting and assessing alignment is like recalibrating your compass to stay on track.

In essence, the implementation is when the rubber meets the road. It's the culmination of your planning efforts and the initiation of tangible progress. Your ability to execute tasks, monitor progress, manage resources, handle issues, and stay aligned with objectives will be instrumental in the successful realization of your health care informatics project.

Maintenance Support of Ongoing Product Development

As you move deeper into the realm of health care informatics, you'll encounter two crucial phases: maintenance support of ongoing product development and a decision to change the product. These phases are integral to the lifecycle of health care systems and require careful consideration.

During maintenance support of ongoing product development, your focus is on maintaining the health of health care informatics products. This involves establishing structured maintenance processes, akin to creating a playbook for product upkeep. It's about ensuring the system remains in optimal condition.

Handling updates and improvements is a vital component. Just as a car needs regular servicing to perform well, health care informatics products require updates and improvements to stay effective. Continuous monitoring is your watchful eye, allowing you to observe how the product functions and gather feedback from users for ongoing enhancements.

Moreover, integration with development is paramount. Imagine it as harmonizing all the moving parts within your health care system. Effective teamwork among development, support, and operations teams is essential to maintain and enhance the product cohesively.

A Decision to Change the Product

On the other hand, a decision to change the product signifies a pivotal juncture. Here, you must articulate the reasons for considering a change. Providing context and clarity to stakeholders is vital for informed decision-making.

Conducting an impact assessment is your compass in helping you navigate potential changes. You'll evaluate how modifications may affect various aspects, including costs, resources, and project timelines. Inclusivity is key; involving stakeholders ensures that decisions are well-rounded and supported.

Once a decision is reached, it's time to plan how the change will be implemented. This involves defining steps, assigning responsibilities, and ensuring a seamless transition. Effective communication throughout the process ensures that all stakeholders are informed and aligned.

By following these steps diligently, you equip yourself to handle strategic planning, project management, and product changes adeptly within an organization. Each stage contributes to a well-rounded understanding, fostering a seamless and successful journey toward achieving your organizational goals in the dynamic field of health care informatics.

Illustration of the Process and Steps

Let's look at two hypothetical cases to illustrate the steps in the process related to telehealth in patient care, with a focus on the role of an informaticist. In case one, you'll follow Nurse Emily Williams, an informaticist, as she navigates the process.

Case 1: Enhancing Telehealth Services in a Healthcare Facility

Step 1: Strategic Information Plan

Nurse Emily Williams works as the chief informaticist at E-Health Medical Center. The organization's long-term goal is to improve patient access to health care services, especially in remote areas. Nurse Williams identifies this as the first step in their strategic information plan.

> *Identification of long-term organizational goals and objectives*: The primary goal is to expand telehealth services to reach underserved areas.
>
> *Assessment of IT's contribution*: Nurse Williams assesses how telehealth technology can bridge the gap by connecting patients and health care providers remotely.
>
> *Definition of strategies*: She formulates strategies to acquire advanced telehealth technology, manage patient data securely, and utilize resources efficiently.
>
> *Alignment with business strategy*: Nurse Williams ensures that the telehealth plan aligns with E-Health's mission of providing accessible health care.
>
> *Consideration of technology trends*: She stays updated on the latest telehealth innovations and identifies potential risks, such as data security concerns.

Step 2: Tactical Information Plan

Nurse Williams moves on to the tactical plan, breaking down the strategic goals into actionable steps.

Detailed plans and actions: She creates a step-by-step plan, outlining how to implement and scale up telehealth services.

Technology specifications: Nurse Williams selects the necessary telehealth platforms, including videoconferencing tools, EHR systems, and secure messaging platforms.

Budget allocation: She estimates the budget required for equipment, software, and staff training.

Timeline for implementation: Nurse Williams sets deadlines for different phases of the telehealth rollout.

User training and communication: She designs training programs for health care staff and develops patient communication materials explaining the new telehealth services.

Step 3: Principles of Project Management & Organization Management

Nurse Williams ensures the project follows established project management principles.

Introduction to project management: She briefs her team on project management concepts, emphasizing the importance of scope, time, and cost management.

Key project management principles: Nurse Williams emphasizes quality, ensuring that the telehealth system is user-friendly and reliable.

Various methodologies: She chooses an Agile approach to allow flexibility in adapting to changing patient needs.

Integration within the organization: Nurse Williams integrates telehealth workflows into existing health care processes.

Leadership and communication: She leads her team, emphasizing regular communication to address issues and maintain stakeholder engagement.

Step 4: System Selection Task Force

Nurse Williams assembles a task force to evaluate and select the most suitable telehealth system.

Formation and composition: The task force includes IT experts, clinicians, and patient representatives.

Identification of needs: They identify that the system should support video consultations, secure data transfer, and remote monitoring.

Evaluation criteria: The task force develops criteria such as ease of use, data security, and scalability.

Evaluation and comparison: They assess several telehealth platforms, comparing features and costs.

Decision-making process: After thorough evaluation, they select a comprehensive telehealth solution that meets the organization's needs.

Step 5: Agreement on the Scope of the Project

To ensure a clear and structured approach to expanding telehealth services, Nurse Williams and her team establish key project scope elements, including the following:

Detailed project description: Nurse Williams and her team create a project description that outlines the expansion of telehealth services to cover remote areas, emphasizing primary care and mental health.

Project deliverables: They specify that the deliverables include a fully functional telehealth infrastructure, staff training, and patient education materials.

Scope boundaries: The team defines what's included (telehealth services) and excluded (major infrastructure changes).

Roles and responsibilities: Nurse Williams assigns responsibilities to team members for different aspects of the project.

Change-control processes: They develop a process for managing any changes or deviations from the original scope.

Step 6: Finalization of Project Details

As Nurse Williams moves into Step 6, Finalization of Project Details, her focus shifts to ensuring every aspect of her plan is finely tuned and ready for execution. The key activities involved in this phase are:

Refinement of plans: The team refines the implementation schedule and allocates resources.

Resource allocation: Nurse Williams assigns tasks and secures necessary resources, including personnel and equipment.

Comprehensive project plan document: They create a detailed project plan, ensuring everyone has access to it.

Risk assessment: Nurse Williams identifies potential risks, such as technical glitches and patient adoption issues, and plans mitigation strategies.

Communication plan: A communication plan is developed to keep stakeholders informed about project progress.

Step 7: Implementing the Project

The project kicks off, with Nurse Williams overseeing the execution of the plan.

Execution of tasks: The telehealth infrastructure is set up, staff is trained, and patient education materials are distributed.

Monitoring progress: Regular check-ins ensure that the project stays on track.

Resource and budget management: Nurse Williams ensures that resources are used efficiently.

Issue management: She addresses technical problems promptly and adjusts the plan if needed.

Alignment with objectives: Throughout the implementation, Nurse Williams keeps an eye on whether the project aligns with the organization's goals.

Step 8: Maintenance Support of Ongoing Product Development

After the telehealth system is operational, Nurse Williams establishes ongoing maintenance processes.

Maintenance processes: The project team establish procedures for updating software, monitoring performance, and addressing patient feedback.

Handling updates and improvements: Nurse Williams oversees the integration of new features and improvements into the telehealth system.

Continuous monitoring: Regularly reviewing performance metrics and patient feedback helps the project team maintain quality.

Integration with development: Maintenance activities are seamlessly integrated with the organization's development cycles.

Collaboration: Nurse Williams fosters collaboration among IT, clinical, and support teams to ensure the telehealth system runs smoothly.

Step 9: A Decision to Change the Product

As technology evolves, Nurse Williams and her team consider improvements to the telehealth system.

Reasons for change: They identify that the current telehealth system needs updates to incorporate AI-driven diagnostic tools and enhanced patient engagement features.

Impact assessment: They assess the costs, resource requirements, and timeline for implementing these changes.

Decision-making process: Nurse Williams involves stakeholders in the decision to upgrade the telehealth system.

Change management plan: A plan is developed to implement the upgrades seamlessly.

Communication strategy: They prepare to announce the changes to both staff and patients, ensuring a smooth transition.

Throughout this hypothetical case, Nurse Emily Williams demonstrates how an informaticist can play a crucial role in developing and implementing telehealth services while aligning them with organizational goals and ensuring ongoing quality and improvement.

Case 2

Imagine you're a dedicated public health professional working in a community that has been grappling with a serious lead poisoning crisis, much like the Flint, Michigan, water crisis. You're deeply concerned about the long-term health and well-being of the residents, especially the children, who are most vulnerable to the effects of lead exposure. To address this critical issue, you decide to embark on a project that will educate the community about lead poisoning and provide essential support to affected families.

Step 1: Initiation

The first step is to initiate the project. In this case, it involves creating a digital registration form to capture important data, such as household income. This initiation phase would involve identifying the need for such a form, its purpose, and the benefits it would bring in terms of gathering relevant information efficiently. You realize that understanding the community's economic status is crucial for tailoring your educational efforts and support programs effectively.

Step 2: Planning

Once the need is established, you need to plan the project. This involves conducting research on lead poisoning, which will inform the content for a YouTube video. Planning also includes defining the scope of the video's target audience (the community, with a focus on children) and the sequence of long-term care that will be presented in the video. Additionally, you should plan for periodic follow-ups after the video release. Your goal is to create a comprehensive educational resource that addresses the specific needs of your community.

Step 3: Execution

With the planning in place, you move on to the execution phase. This phase includes reaching out to a family impacted by the crisis and setting up videoconferencing for that family. It also involves creating the YouTube video based on the research conducted earlier. The goal is to provide educational content to the community that is both informative and empathetic, helping them understand the severity of the issue and the available resources for support.

Step 4: Monitoring and Control

Throughout the project, you need to monitor progress and make any necessary adjustments. For example, you should regularly check the video's performance on YouTube and gather feedback from the community to see if it's effectively educating them about lead poisoning. If necessary, you can make improvements to the video or its distribution strategy. This ensures that your educational efforts remain effective and relevant.

Step 5: Closure

Once the video is in place and has been shared with the community, it's important to set goals with the family impacted by the situation. These goals will address their specific needs and concerns related to lead poisoning. Additionally, creating a website to give virtual/mobile access to you and the information prepared for them is part of the closure phase, as it ensures ongoing support and access to resources. It's about ensuring that the knowledge and support provided during the project continue to benefit the community.

Step 6: Maintenance and Enhancement

After the initial project is completed, it's essential to maintain and enhance the educational efforts. This includes creating additional content, such as educational humor videos that reinforce the idea that access to care will always be available. It also involves keeping the website up-to-date and responsive to the evolving needs of the community. This ongoing commitment ensures that your efforts to combat lead poisoning remain effective and sustainable.

By following this system life cycle approach, you can systematically plan, execute, and sustain your efforts to educate the community about lead poisoning and provide support to affected families. Your dedication and structured approach can make a significant difference in improving the health and well-being of the community you serve.

Hello!
My name is
Dr. Clear Water

Meet
The Flintwater
Team
Ms. Magic Meals
Filterman

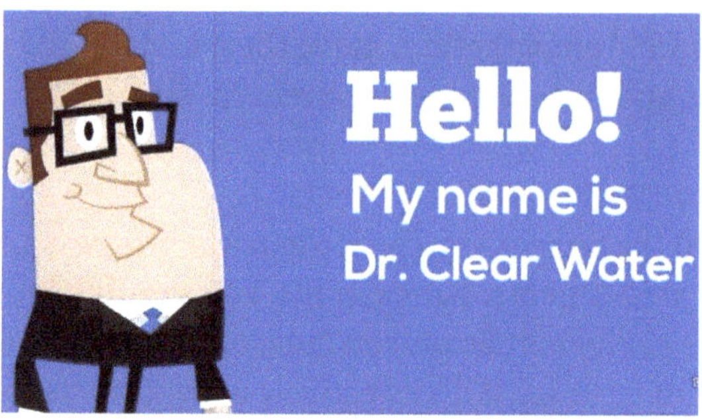

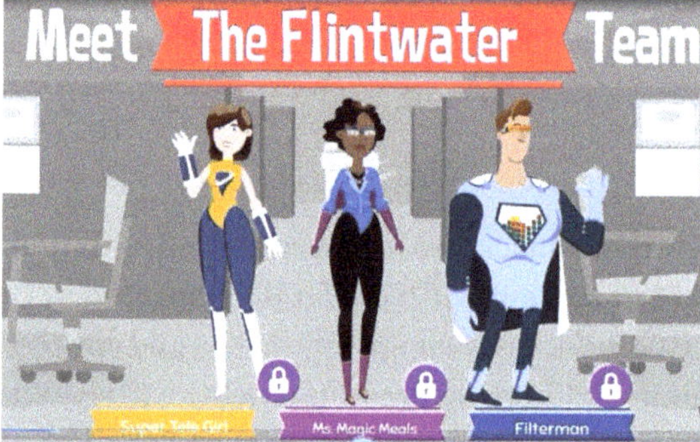

FIGURE 5.2 Charting the course with a touch of humor.

Summary

In this chapter, we embarked on a journey through the intricate world of HIS. From understanding the HIS life cycle to delving deep into the principles of project management and organization, we've gained valuable insights into the critical systems that drive modern health care.

In this chapter, you bridged the gap between theory and practice, equipping yourself with the knowledge needed to navigate HIS projects successfully. You explored the essential steps, strategic decisions, and the often-overlooked aspects of ongoing product development and post-launch support. This knowledge is your compass as you journey through the dynamic landscape of health care informatics.

You covered concepts ranging from strategy and tactics to assembling project teams, defining scopes, employing fast-track methods, and making pivotal change decisions. These elements constitute the core of effective HIS project management, ensuring success in an ever-evolving health care environment.

But there's more to discover. Decision-making within health care organizations can lead to significant changes in the products you design and bring to life. These decisions ripple through processes, influence patient care, and shape the health care landscape itself.

As you move forward, keep embracing the challenges and opportunities within the HIS system life cycle. Your understanding of the technical intricacies, coupled with your appreciation for strategic thinking, collaboration, and adaptability, will empower you to make a meaningful impact in the realm of HIS.

Remember that your journey doesn't end here. In your future endeavors, you'll actively contribute to the successful realization and evolution of HIS within the dynamic health care landscape. Case scenarios provided practical insights and hands-on experience, preparing you to navigate the complexities of HCIS effectively.

As you turn the page to the next chapter, carry with you the knowledge, skills, and enthusiasm gained in this chapter. The world of HIS awaits your expertise and innovation, and together, you'll continue to explore the cutting edge of health care informatics.

Chapter Review Questions

Directions: Consider what you learned in this chapter as you respond to the health care scenario and questions.

Health Care Scenario: Implementing a New HIS

You are part of a health care organization that is implementing a new HIS. The goal is to improve patient data management, streamline workflows, and enhance overall care delivery. Your organization has assembled a cross-functional task force to evaluate and select the most suitable HIS system, considering budget constraints and technical requirements. The task force is responsible for defining the project scope, developing a strategic information plan, and ensuring effective project management and organizational principles are applied throughout the project life cycle. The implementation plan includes software and hardware upgrades, staff training, and data security measures. The team must also ensure ongoing maintenance and support postlaunch, addressing user feedback and technological advancements.

Multiple-Choice Questions

1. What is the primary objective of assembling a cross-functional task force for the HIS project?
    a. To increase the workload on staff
    b. To evaluate, select, and recommend the most suitable HIS system
    c. To delay the project timeline
    d. To reduce the overall project budget
2. Which of the following is a key component of the strategic information plan for the HIS project?
    a. Daily staff meetings
    b. Social media marketing
    c. Aligned long-term goals: data management, technology, and resources
    d. Organizing office parties
3. What is the significance of defining the project scope in the HIS project?
    a. To minimize project documentation
    b. To make the project more complex
    c. To ensure clarity and alignment with organizational goals
    d. To eliminate the need for staff training

4. Which method can be used to accelerate the development and deployment of the HIS system while maintaining quality and compliance?
    a. Ignoring quality standards
    b. Reducing the number of staff
    c. Postponing project milestones
    d. Fast-tracking design-and-build methods
5. What should be included in the tactical information plan for HIS implementation?
    a. Short- to medium-term strategies: upgrades, training, security measures
    b. Long-term visions without actionable steps
    c. Hiring social media influencers
    d. Organizing annual health care conferences
6. How should ongoing maintenance and support of the HIS be managed postlaunch?
    a. By ignoring user feedback
    b. By conducting regular updates, bug fixes, and user training
    c. By discontinuing the HIS system after launch
    d. By reducing the IT support team

Answer Key

1. (b) To evaluate, select, and recommend the most suitable HIS system
2. (c) Long-term goals alignment focusing on data management, technology infrastructure, and resource allocation
3. (c) To ensure clarity and alignment with organizational goals
4. (d) Fast-tracking design-and-build methods
5. (a) Short- to medium-term strategies, including software and hardware upgrades, staff training, and data security measures
6. (b) By conducting regular updates, bug fixes, and user training

References

Nelson, R., & Staggers, N. (2014). *Health informatics: An interprofessional approach*. Elsevier.

Wager, K. A., Lee, F. W., & Glaser, J. P. (2022). *Health care information systems: A practical approach for health care management* (5th ed.). Jossey-Bass.

Figure Credits

Fig. 5.2a: Generated using Powtoon.com. Copyright © by Powtoon.com, Inc. Reprinted with permission.

Fig. 5.2b: Generated using Nawmal. Copyright © by Technologies Nawmal, Inc. Reprinted with permission.

Chapter 6

Business Intelligence Techniques and Tools Used for the Transformation of Data Into Meaningful Use and Useful Information for Business

Introduction

The purpose of Chapter 6 is to provide readers with a comprehensive understanding of business intelligence (BI) techniques, vendor selection strategies, and the practical skills necessary for transforming health care data into actionable information. By mastering these concepts, readers will be empowered to make informed decisions and significantly contribute to the decision-making processes within health care organizations. This chapter emphasizes the development of critical thinking and problem-solving skills through engaging discussions and hypothetical scenarios, preparing readers to tackle real-world challenges with effective BI solutions.

Chapter 6 is significant because it equips readers with the expertise needed to navigate and excel in the dynamic field of HIS. The chapter fosters continuous learning and practical application, blending technical knowledge with strategic thinking, collaboration, and adaptability. This holistic approach aims to drive meaningful changes in health care by leveraging BI. The consensus in the literature highlights the crucial role of BI in health care informatics, underscoring its potential to revolutionize the industry. By embracing BI, readers will be at the forefront of ensuring that data-driven decisions become the foundation of health care excellence, ultimately reshaping the landscape and improving patient outcomes.

Throughout this chapter, critical thinking will be your guiding light. Engaging discussions and hypothetical scenarios will promote analytical thinking related to BI in health care. You'll develop problem-solving skills, enabling us to dissect real-world scenarios and propose effective BI solutions.

Remember, your journey is one of continuous learning and practical application. Your expertise in technical nuances, coupled with strategic ingenuity, a collaborative spirit, and adaptability, will be the driving force behind meaningful changes in the realm of HIS. Together, let's embark on this exploration, unraveling the complexities and embracing the innovations that BI brings to the dynamic health care landscape.

Armed with curiosity, determination, and the shared vision of making a difference, let's dive into this mission. Our journey is not just an exploration; it's a mission—a mission to revolutionize health care through the lens of BI. The consensus of literature affirms the significance of BI and the role it plays in health care informatics. With this understanding, we have the potential to reshape the landscape, ensuring that data-driven decisions become the cornerstone of health care excellence.

Objectives That Lead to Outcomes

By clearly distinguishing between process-oriented objectives and result-oriented outcomes, it becomes easier to understand and measure both the actions taken and the results achieved. Thus, the following table aligns key objectives with their corresponding outcomes, providing a clear and detailed understanding of what learners should achieve and comprehend upon completion.

Objective	Outcome
Recognize challenges in health care data management and integration.	Identify data security, quality, compliance issues in health care settings.
Develop strategies for effective BI implementation in health care.	Address data challenges and optimize BI integration.
Evaluate methods for selecting suitable BI vendor products in health care.	Develop criteria for selecting BI tools that enhance health care outcomes and efficiency.
Analyze criteria for evaluating BI tools in health care.	Apply criteria for improved health care outcomes and operational efficiency.
Understand methods for comprehensive evaluation of BI products in health care.	Assess BI product sustainability and suitability for health care environments.
Develop negotiation skills for securing favorable BI vendor contracts in health care.	Secure advantageous contracts with effective negotiation strategies.
Navigate the vendor selection process for BI tools in health care.	Successfully navigate steps from requirements to final vendor selection.
Apply advanced BI techniques to address health care challenges.	Utilize AI, ML, and big data analytics for health care–specific challenges.

Key Terms

Directions: Before reading, please look at this list of key terms that will be used in this chapter. If any term is unfamiliar, please see the glossary at the end of the book.

application of processes
core concepts
critical thought
informatics
key principles
modeling
resource
tangible example pages of the website
theories
website design

Staying on Track: Unraveling Insights

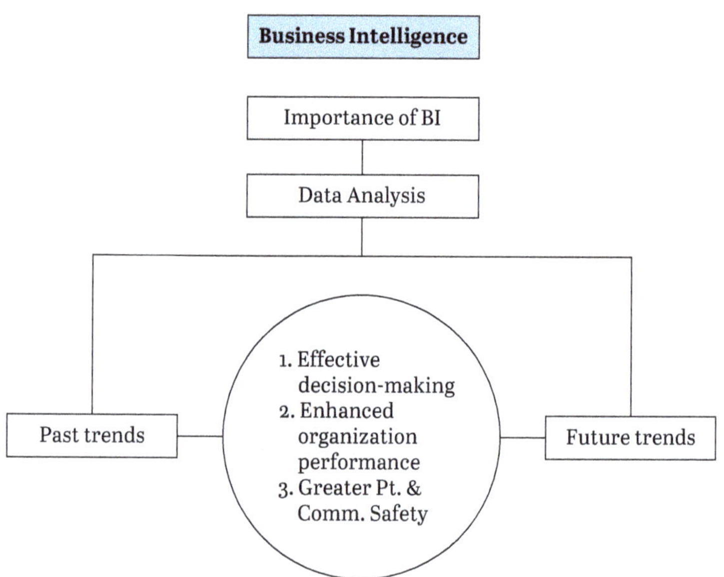

FIGURE 6.1 Making the connections.

Navigating the BI Landscape

In the ever-evolving landscape of health care technology, we've journeyed through the intricate pathways of HIS, understanding their life cycles and the pivotal role they play in modern health care. Just as health care data forms the beating heart of the industry, our exploration has led us to a new frontier: BI.

As we move beyond the stages of collecting, storing, and processing data in the HIS life cycle, we enter the fascinating world of BI. This is when raw data undergoes a remarkable transformation, evolving into a source of incredibly valuable insights. It's a journey from mere information to powerful knowledge, and it's a pivotal step in understanding how data truly shapes decisions and strategies in various fields, including health care. Think of BI as the magic of the digital age, whereby the power lies in the methods and tools employed to transmute raw data into meaningful, actionable intelligence

(El-Gayar & Timsina, 2014). Chapter 5 was a voyage into the heart of the HIS, and data integrity and accessibility were paramount. In this chapter, we shift our focus to the strategic implementation of BI techniques and tools. These not only refine data, but also illuminate patterns, trends, and opportunities hidden within its vast expanse. We explore the very essence of BI: the art and science of turning data into decisions.

Navigating Data Challenges in Health Care Informatics

Health care informatics presents numerous challenges that impact the success of organizations. BI, first introduced by Richard Miller Devens in 1865, has influenced the industry for over 150 years (Lago, 2018). Organizations must continuously address issues related to data security, quality, compliance, and integration to ensure effective BI implementation.

TABLE 6.1 Analytics in Use

Data-Mining Process	Analytics Process	Analytic Steps
1. Collect and integrate data: Gather a cluster of data from various sources. 2. Organize and prepare data: Structure and organize data for analysis. 3. Select and transform data: Identify useful data for mining. 4. Apply data mining algorithms: Employ algorithms to build predictive and descriptive models.	1. Understand the meaning for application: Grasp the context and purpose for analysis. 2. Develop descriptive and analytical models: Create models for in-depth analysis and insight generation.	1. *Define objectives and dataset selection*: Clearly outline goals and choose appropriate dataset. 2. Data preparation and processing: Prepare data and process it for analysis. 3. Manipulation and analysis of datasets: Explore and analyze data, seeking patterns for description and prediction.

A thorough understanding of these challenges provides a foundation for leveraging BI in health care informatics. Historical context, coupled with current complexities, highlights the critical role of secure and reliable data in decision-making. Addressing these issues paves the way for advanced analytics, including data mining techniques that extract meaningful patterns from large datasets. Examining each step of the analytical process reveals how raw data is transformed into actionable intelligence.

Seamlessly integrating these elements offers a comprehensive perspective on health care informatics. Overcoming data challenges enables organizations to maximize the potential of analytics, driving informed decisions and improving patient outcomes.

Understanding Common Challenges

Data Security

Health care organizations handle sensitive patient data, making them lucrative targets for cyber threats. Ensuring robust data encryption, access controls, and regular security audits is imperative to safeguard patient confidentiality and comply with regulations such as HIPAA (Health Insurance Portability and Accountability Act).

Data Quality

The accuracy and reliability of health care data are pivotal for informed decision-making. Challenges arise from data silos, inconsistent formats, and human errors. Implementing data governance frameworks, standardizing protocols, and investing in data cleansing tools enhance data quality.

Compliance

Navigating the complex landscape of health care regulations, like the Health Information Technology for Economic and Clinical Health Act, demands meticulous attention. Organizations must establish stringent protocols for adherence, including regular audits, staff training, and staying abreast of evolving compliance requirements.

Data Integration

Health care facilities often utilize diverse systems that don't seamlessly communicate. This siloed approach impedes efficient data exchange. Integration solutions, like Health Level Seven International standards and application programming interfaces, bridge disparate systems, enabling seamless data flow.

Key Strategies for Effective Resolution

Promoting Data Security

Organizations must invest in advanced cybersecurity measures, conduct regular employee training, and establish incident response protocols. Collaborating with cybersecurity experts ensures the development of robust defense mechanisms against evolving threats.

Enhancing Data Quality

Implementing data governance policies, employing data stewards, and utilizing master data management tools standardize data formats, ensuring consistency. Regular audits and feedback loops refine data quality processes, making them more efficient over time.

Ensuring Compliance

Continuous education, coupled with robust compliance management software, aids in keeping track of regulatory changes. Regular internal audits and collaborations with legal experts guarantee that the organization's practices align with the latest health care regulations.

Facilitating Data Integration

Adopting interoperability standards and investing in middleware solutions facilitate seamless data exchange. Collaboration with system developers and IT experts helps customize integration methods according to organizational needs.

Selecting Suitable Vendor Products

Comprehensive Needs Assessment

Prior to vendor selection, organizations must conduct an in-depth analysis of their requirements. Identifying specific needs, such as scalability, customization, and support, guides the selection process.

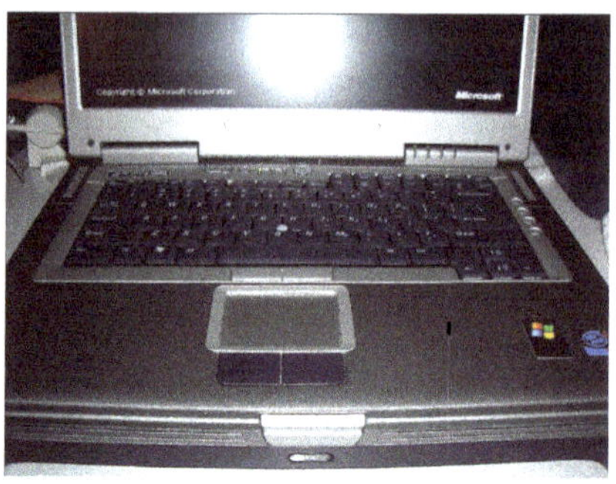

FIGURE 6.2 Vendor selection: Compatibility is key.

Vendor Reputation and Expertise

Researching vendor track records, customer testimonials, and case studies provide insights into their competence. Engaging with vendors directly through demonstrations and consultations gauges their understanding of health care informatics challenges.

Scalability and Compatibility

The chosen product should not only meet current needs but also scale with the organization's growth. Compatibility with existing systems and future technologies ensures a seamless integration process.

Health care informatics' challenges are diverse and demanding. Addressing data security, quality, compliance, and integration issues requires a multifaceted approach. By implementing robust strategies and selecting suitable vendor products, health care organizations can navigate these challenges effectively, ensuring the seamless implementation of BI solutions for informed decision-making and improved patient outcomes.

As we delve into the intricacies of health care informatics challenges and strategies to overcome them, it's crucial to bridge your understanding to the evaluation of BI tools. Evaluating these tools is not just a technical necessity; it's a strategic move with far-reaching implications on health care outcomes, cost-effectiveness, and operational efficiency.

In our quest to enhance patient care, we must meticulously assess BI tools based on their potential to improve health care outcomes. An effective tool should provide actionable insights derived from data analysis, empowering health care professionals to make informed decisions that directly impact patient well-being. Simultaneously, we can't overlook the financial aspect. A tool's cost-effectiveness is pivotal, ensuring that valuable resources are utilized optimally, making advanced health care technology accessible without burdening budgets.

Amid this evaluation, the importance of sustainability looms large. Sustainable BI tools ensure long-term usability, aligning with evolving health care needs and technological advancements. Learning methods for comprehensive product evaluation equips us with the ability to foresee the tool's viability over time. Sustainability isn't just about the software's life span; it's about how well it adapts to the ever-changing landscape of health care.

Now, armed with a profound understanding of evaluation criteria and sustainability, we pivot to the practical aspect of navigating the vendor selection process. This journey is more than just choosing a product; it's about honing negotiation skills and strategies that are indispensable in securing favorable contracts with BI vendors.

Negotiation in this context isn't merely a transactional dialogue; it's a collaborative process. It's about understanding the vendor's perspective while safeguarding the interests of our health care organization. Developing negotiation skills isn't just about haggling over prices; it's about ensuring that the contract is comprehensive, covering aspects such as support, updates, and scalability.

In the vendor selection process, every step is crucial. From the initial needs assessment to the final contract signing, it's a continuum on which our understanding of product evaluation criteria, sustainability, and negotiation skills converge. It's about making informed decisions that resonate with your organization's goals, ensuring that the chosen BI tool becomes an asset, propelling us toward a future when health care outcomes are optimized, costs are managed efficiently, and operations run seamlessly.

As we navigate these challenges and strategies, let's remember that our journey doesn't end with overcoming obstacles; it extends to choosing the right tools and partners that will shape the future of health care informatics, ultimately enhancing patient care and transforming health care delivery.

Navigating the Intersection

Technical Evaluation, Contract Negotiation, and Scope Definition in Health Care Informatics

Having navigated the intricacies of vendor selection and contract negotiation, our journey in health care informatics propels us into the realm of technical evaluation. It's not just about choosing a product; it's about selecting the right product tailored to our health care-specific requirements. Techniques to assess and compare vendor products in the context of health care are multifaceted. We delve deep into the functionalities that directly impact patient care, such as predictive analytics for early disease detection or real-time data processing for critical patient monitoring.

Yet, even with the perfect product, the intricacies of contract negotiation continue. It's not merely about hammering out terms; it's about ensuring flexibility for future upgrades. In the rapidly evolving landscape of health care technology, the ability to adapt and incorporate new features is paramount. Simultaneously, we must be vigilant about legal risks, ensuring that our organization is protected from potential liabilities.

With contracts solidified, our focus shifts to the foundational stage of any BI project: defining its scope. This phase is pivotal, aligning the project with our organizational objectives. It's about asking the right questions: What health care challenges are we solving? How does this align with our mission to enhance patient care? Defining the scope isn't just a technicality; it's the blueprint that guides the entire project, ensuring that every effort contributes meaningfully to our organizational goals.

In the intricate web of project details lies the key to successful implementation. It's not just about the technical aspects; it's about understanding the pulse of our organization. It's about collaboration, communication, and consensus. This phase demands meticulous planning, addressing every nuance, and foreseeing potential roadblocks. It's about ensuring that our vision aligns seamlessly with the technical capabilities of our chosen BI tool.

Yet, the journey doesn't end here; it transforms. Armed with a comprehensive understanding of our organizational needs, a well-negotiated contract, and a meticulously defined project scope, we transition into the application phase. This is when theory meets reality. We apply the acquired BI techniques to real health care challenges. This is about using predictive analytics to anticipate disease outbreaks, optimizing resource allocation for maximum efficiency, and harnessing the power of data to enhance patient experiences.

In this journey, each step is interlinked, forming a continuum on which knowledge, strategy, and implementation converge. It's not just about mastering the tools; it's about understanding the heartbeat of health care, whereby technology becomes a catalyst for transformative change. As we progress, let's remember that our endeavors in health care informatics are not just academic exercises; they are real-world solutions, shaping the future of health care one data point at a time. This transition connects the discussion on evaluating vendor products, contract negotiation, defining project scope, and applying BI techniques, emphasizing the practical application of knowledge to solve health care challenges.

Having mastered the foundational aspects of BI, our journey propels us into the realm of practical application. It's here that theory transforms into transformative action. Armed with a comprehensive understanding of BI techniques, including AI, ML, and big data analytics, we delve deep into the heart of health care challenges.

In the intricate landscape of health care entities, challenges abound. Improving patient care isn't just a slogan; it's a tangible goal that we can achieve through the strategic application of these advanced techniques. AI empowers us to predict patient outcomes, providing timely interventions that can be life-saving. Machine-learning algorithms analyze vast datasets, identifying patterns that human eyes might miss, leading to more accurate diagnoses and personalized treatment plans.

Resource allocation, a critical concern in any health care organization, becomes a nuanced art when guided by data-driven insights. BI techniques enable us to optimize resources, ensuring that every dollar and every minute is utilized to its fullest potential. By identifying trends in patient admissions, treatment outcomes, and operational inefficiencies, we can make informed decisions that not only improve patient experiences, but also streamline internal processes.

Cost reduction, a perpetual challenge, finds its solution in the judicious use of big data analytics. By analyzing the cost-effectiveness of different treatments, medications, and procedures, we can identify areas for which costs can be minimized without compromising the quality of care. It's not just about cutting expenses; it's about doing so strategically, ensuring that every cost-cutting measure contributes positively to patient outcomes.

Visual Mastery

Transforming Data Into Compelling Narratives in BI

These applications aren't isolated efforts; they are interconnected threads in the tapestry of health care transformation. As we apply BI techniques to solve specific health care challenges, we are not just processing data; we are enhancing lives. Every accurate diagnosis, every streamlined process, and every optimized resource allocation decision directly impacts patients, making their health care journey smoother, more efficient, and ultimately more compassionate.

In this phase of our learning journey, we become architects of change, utilizing advanced BI techniques as our tools. Each technique isn't just a line of code or an algorithm; it's a potential solution to a health care challenge. As we immerse ourselves in this hands-on experience, let's remember that our efforts are not just academic exercises; they are building blocks of a healthier, more efficient, and more patient-centric health care system. Our understanding and application of these advanced techniques aren't just skills; they are catalysts for a brighter, healthier future.

Visualizing Complexity

Bridging Understanding in BI Communication

As we navigate the dynamic landscape of health care informatics, we encounter a pivotal aspect of modern communication: the art of visual representation. Words and data, no matter how precise, often find their true power when translated into visuals. This transformative process is not just about creating PowerPoint presentations; it's about mastering the art of blending aesthetics with information.

Ferranti et al. (2010) supports the notion that in the realm of BI, in which data can be vast and complex, the ability to translate intricate processes into understandable visuals is a valuable skill. Imagine crafting a flowchart that simplifies a convoluted data analysis process or designing a graph that vividly illustrates trends and patterns. These visuals transcend mere images; they become powerful tools of communication, conveying complex concepts with clarity.

When we delve into the creation of PowerPoint presentations, we're not just arranging slides; we're crafting narratives. Infographics become our storytelling companions, distilling vast datasets into comprehensible snippets. The interplay of colors, shapes, and data points isn't just artistic expression; it's a method to enhance understanding. It's about transforming raw information into compelling stories that resonate with the audience, be it colleagues, stakeholders, or patients.

Yet, the significance of visual representation extends beyond aesthetics. It's a fundamental aspect of effective communication. In the context of BI, visual representations serve as bridges between technical jargon and practical insights. They transform abstract numbers into tangible narratives, enabling stakeholders to grasp the nuances of BI concepts and outcomes intuitively.

In essence, our venture into creating visual representations is not just a creative endeavor; it's a strategic one. It's about translating the language of data into a universal dialect that speaks to everyone. As we continue to embark on this journey, let's remember that these visuals aren't just slides; they are gateways to understanding. They are bridges that connect the complexity of BI processes with the clarity of comprehension. Each visual representation we create isn't just an image; it's a conduit for knowledge, paving the way for a deeper understanding of the transformative power of BI in health care.

Empowering Change

As you approach the culmination of your journey in health care informatics, there's a pivotal shift in focus: from acquiring knowledge to honing critical thinking and problem-solving skills. It's not just about what you know; it's about how you apply that knowledge in real-world scenarios.

In the realm of BI, critical thinking becomes your guiding light. You engage in discussions and delve into case studies that challenge you to analyze complex situations. You dissect real-world scenarios, identifying nuances, challenges, and opportunities. Through this process, you don't just find answers; you cultivate the art of asking the right questions. You learn to probe deeper, challenge assumptions, and explore uncharted territories of thought.

Problem-solving also becomes second nature. Armed with your knowledge of BI, you propose solutions that are not mere theoretical constructs but pragmatic pathways to success. You bridge the gap between problems and solutions, using data-driven insights to inform your decisions. You learn that problem-solving isn't a linear process; it's an iterative journey, and each attempt refines your understanding and sharpens your skills.

Your learning journey doesn't halt here; it transforms into a continuous cycle of growth. You embrace the concept of lifelong learning, understanding that in the realm of BI, stagnation is not an option. The field evolves, and so must you. You stay updated with the latest trends and technologies, not just as a formality but as a necessity. You adapt your strategies, aligning them with the ever-changing landscape of health care.

This adaptability isn't just a skill; it's a mindset. It's about being agile, anticipating challenges before they arise, and proactively seeking innovative solutions. As you step into real-world health care settings, your goal isn't just to apply your knowledge; it's to make a difference. You immerse yourself in the practical application of BI techniques, understanding that your actions have a direct impact on patient care, operational efficiency, and the overall health care ecosystem.

In this final phase, you don't just graduate with a set of skills; you graduate with a mindset—a mindset of continuous learning, critical thinking, and proactive problem-solving. You become an architect of change, equipped not just to navigate the challenges of today but to anticipate and shape the solutions of tomorrow. As you venture into the professional world, remember that your journey doesn't end here; it transforms into a legacy, and the seeds of your learning sprout into innovations that redefine the future of health care through the lens of BI.

This smooth transition emphasizes the importance of fostering critical thinking and problem-solving skills, encouraging continuous learning, and promoting the practical application of BI techniques in real-world health care settings. It highlights the transformative nature of learning, transitioning from acquiring knowledge to shaping a mindset of adaptability, innovation, and proactive problem-solving.

Scenario

Optimizing Patient Care With BI

In a bustling urban hospital, the health care team faced a significant challenge: managing patient care efficiently while maintaining high-quality standards. The hospital implemented BI techniques to address this issue.

Vendor Selection and Contract Negotiation

The hospital's IT department meticulously evaluated various vendors, considering their offerings in predictive analytics, real-time monitoring, and data visualization tools. After careful negotiations, they selected a vendor whose system was adaptable, ensuring future upgrades and legal protections were in place.

Defining Project Scope and Critical Thinking

The hospital's health care executives defined the project scope, aligning it with the hospital's mission to enhance patient care. Critical thinking came into play as they analyzed complex patient data. By asking the right questions and exploring nuances in the data, they identified areas for improvement.

Visual Representation and Communication

Using BI tools, the team transformed intricate patient data into visually appealing and informative infographics. These visuals helped health care providers easily grasp trends, enabling them to make data-driven decisions efficiently. The use of clear visuals bridged the gap between technical jargon and practical insights, enhancing communication among stakeholders.

Problem Solving and Adaptability

When challenges arose, the team leveraged problem-solving skills honed through BI training. By iteratively analyzing data and proposing pragmatic solutions, they optimized resource allocation and streamlined patient care workflows. This adaptability mindset ensured they could adjust strategies based on evolving health care trends.

Continuous Learning and Innovation

As the hospital staff immersed themselves in the practical application of BI techniques, they embraced continuous learning. By staying updated with the latest technologies and trends, they proactively sought innovative solutions. This proactive approach led to the development of a customized patient care model, improving both efficiency and patient outcomes.

In this scenario, the integration of BI techniques empowered the health care team to transform challenges into opportunities. By fostering critical thinking, effective communication, and adaptability, they not only enhanced patient care, but also laid the foundation for ongoing innovations in health care informatics.

Summary

Chapter 6 explores the critical role of continuous learning, innovation, and problem-solving in health care informatics. It emphasizes the shift from merely acquiring knowledge to applying critical thinking and data-driven decision-making in real-world health care settings. Through case studies and discussions, students engage in analyzing complex scenarios, challenging assumptions, and developing practical solutions using BI tools.

The chapter also underscores the importance of lifelong learning and adaptability in the rapidly evolving field of health informatics. Staying informed about emerging trends and technologies is essential for driving meaningful improvements in patient care and operational efficiency. Students are encouraged to cultivate a proactive mindset, embracing change as a pathway to innovation and excellence in health care.

By the end of the chapter, students gain a deeper understanding of how strategic thinking, problem-solving, and innovation empower them to become leaders of change, ensuring that health informatics continues to evolve to meet the needs of modern health care systems.

Chapter Review Questions

Directions: Consider what you learned in this chapter as you respond to the health care scenario and questions.

Health Care Scenario: BI Techniques and Tools

You are a BI consultant hired by HealthyLife Hospital, a large health care organization, to improve their data management and decision-making processes. HealthyLife Hospital faces several challenges, including data integration issues, suboptimal vendor selection processes, and the need for advanced BI techniques to enhance patient care and operational efficiency. The hospital's leadership is keen on leveraging BI to improve outcomes, reduce costs, and make data-driven decisions. Your task is to develop a comprehensive BI strategy, select the right BI tools, and implement solutions that address these challenges.

Multiple-Choice Questions

1. HealthyLife Hospital struggles with integrating data from multiple sources, leading to inconsistencies and inefficiencies. Which strategy would best address this challenge?
    a. Implementing data encryption protocols
    b. Selecting vendor products based solely on cost
    c. Developing a centralized data warehouse
    d. Using manual data entry for accuracy
2. To ensure a successful BI implementation, which of the following should be prioritized?
    a. Choosing the vendor with the most advanced features
    b. Aligning the BI project scope with the hospital's organizational goals
    c. Focusing solely on short-term gains
    d. Ignoring staff training requirements
3. When evaluating BI tools, which criterion is most important for improving patient outcomes and operational efficiency?
    a. Evaluating the vendor's marketing strategy
    b. Analyzing how well the tool supports real-time data analytics and decision-making
    c. Choosing tools with the most attractive user interface
    d. Assessing the tool's popularity in the market

4. Which method would be most effective in negotiating favorable contracts with BI vendors for HealthyLife Hospital?
    a. Accepting the initial offer without negotiations
    b. Focusing on long-term partnerships
    c. Developing negotiation skills and strategies
    d. Selecting the cheapest option available
5. To address specific health care challenges such as improving patient care and reducing costs, which advanced BI technique should be applied?
    a. Utilizing ML to predict patient outcomes and optimize resource allocation
    b. Manually analyzing patient records
    c. Relying on traditional spreadsheets
    d. Ignoring historical data trends
6. HealthyLife Hospital needs to evaluate the sustainability of a BI product. Which approach should they take?
    a. Choose the first product they find.
    b. Assess the product's ability to scale and adapt to future health care needs.
    c. Ignore vendor support and updates.
    d. Focus solely on current capabilities.

Answer Key

1. (c) Developing a centralized data warehouse to consolidate data from all sources
2. (b) Aligning the BI project scope with the hospital's organizational goals
3. (b) Analyzing how well the tool supports real-time data analytics and decision-making
4. (c) Developing negotiation skills and strategies
5. (a) Utilizing ML to predict patient outcomes and optimize resource allocation
6. (b) Assess the product's ability to scale and adapt to future health care needs.

Recommended Reading

Sewell, J., & Thede, L. Q. (2013). *Informatics and nursing: Opportunities and challenges* (4th ed.). Lippincott Williams.

Thede, Q.L, & Sewell, J. P. (2009) *Informatics and nursing competencies and applications* (3rd ed.). Wolters Kluwer/Lippincott Williams & Wilkins.

Zhang, C., & Liu, Z. (2019). Application of big data technology in agricultural Internet of Things. *International Journal of Distributed Sensor Networks, 15*(10). https://doi.org/10.1177/1550147719881610

References

El-Gayar, O., & Timsina, P. (2014). *Opportunities for business intelligence and big data analytics in evidence based medicine* [Paper presentation]. 47th Hawaii International Conference on System Sciences, Waikoloa, HI, USA. https://doi.org/10.1109/HICSS.2014.100

Ferranti, J. M., Langman, M. K., Tanaka, D., McCall, J., & Ahmad, A. (2010). Bridging the gap: Leveraging business intelligence tools in support of patient safety and financial effectiveness. *Journal of the American Medical Informatics Association, 17*(2), 136–43. https://doi.org/10.1136/jamia.2009.002220

Lago, C. (2018, July 18). *150 years of business intelligence: A brief history*. CIO. https://www.cio.com/article/221963/history-of-business-intelligence.html

Chapter 7

Exploring the Possibilities of Telehealth

A Comprehensive Guide

Introduction

The purpose of Chapter 7 is to transition from knowledge acquisition to the development of critical thinking and problem-solving skills within health care informatics. It examines telehealth approaches in clinical practice, education, and community care, focusing on practical applications. The chapter explores how telehealth, mobile health, and health information networks (HINs) can be effectively implemented across various settings, including office-based practices, homecare, and public health.

The significance of Chapter 7 lies in its role in bridging the gap between theoretical knowledge and practical application in health care informatics. By emphasizing the enhancement of critical thinking, the chapter highlights the importance of utilizing telehealth technologies to improve health care delivery. It explores diverse telehealth scenarios, demonstrating how health care professionals can transform their knowledge into actionable insights. This practical focus ensures that learners are prepared to apply telehealth innovations effectively, fostering positive changes in clinical practice, education, and community health.

As we continue our health care informatics journey, there's a notable shift from knowledge acquisition to the refinement of critical thinking and problem-solving skills. The focus transitions from what we know to how we apply that knowledge in real-world scenarios. In the realm of BI, critical thinking serves as our guiding light. This chapter takes us from office-based settings to the specifics of homecare and the broader landscape of public health. Our journey now involves navigating the diverse landscape of telehealth scenarios, mirroring the overarching theme of transforming knowledge into actionable insights for positive change in health care.

Figure 7.1 serves as an early representation of the profound advantages offered by telehealth, prompting us to envision how we might craft a telehealth strategy that caters to the evolving needs of our society. The visual encapsulates a transformative scenario in which a patient can receive specialized care from experts worldwide without the need to travel beyond their community. This is made possible through a seamless integration of virtual mobile communication. In the depiction, a patient communicates with a specialist located in another country using a mobile device, breaking down geographical barriers. The elimination of air transport is symbolized, underlining the accessibility of specialized care without the logistical challenges of travel. The image further emphasizes the ability to share crucial lab documents with the specialist, ensuring a comprehensive exchange of information.

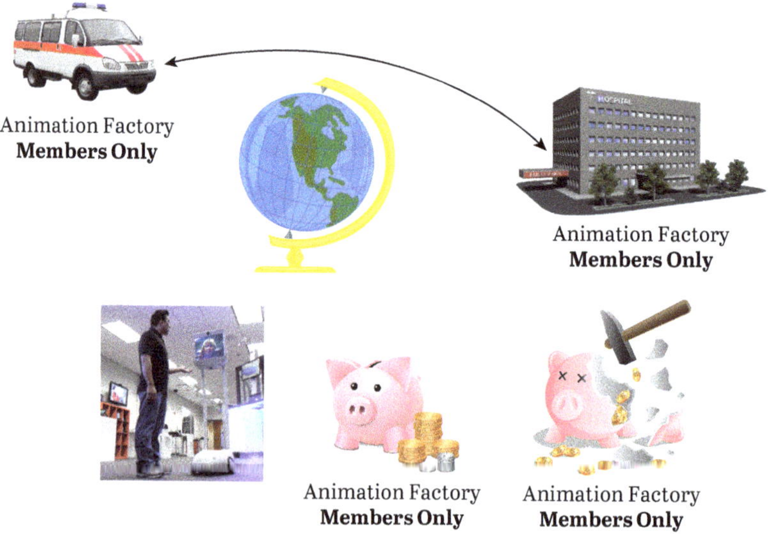

FIGURE 7.1 Telehealth practice making a difference.

Within this visual narrative, the presence of piggy banks strategically placed conveys a subtle yet powerful message of cost-effectiveness. The innovative telehealth approach not only enhances accessibility but also proves to be economically prudent, as illustrated by the piggy banks. This vivid portrayal signifies a landscape ripe with opportunities for innovation in health care. It challenges us to think creatively, inspiring the development of telehealth solutions that can truly revolutionize the way we deliver and receive medical care.

Objectives That Lead to Outcomes

By clearly distinguishing between process-oriented objectives and result-oriented outcomes, it becomes easier to understand and measure both the actions taken and the results achieved. Thus, the following table aligns key objectives with their corresponding outcomes, providing a clear and detailed understanding of what learners should achieve and comprehend upon completion. This alignment ensures that each objective is met with a tangible and measurable outcome, enhancing the overall learning experience.

Objective	Outcome
Analyze the evolution and integration of telehealth, mobile health, and HINs from the 1950s to the present across varied health care settings to enhance patient care and accessibility.	Identify and implement effective telehealth and mobile health strategies that improve patient access and care coordination across different health care settings.
Chart the transformative landscape of telehealth and HINs, evaluating the impact and effectiveness of telehealth and mobile health applications in homecare to improve patient outcomes and the overall quality of health care services delivered.	Demonstrate improved patient outcomes and quality of care in homecare settings through the use of telehealth and mobile health applications.
Assess the role and significance of telehealth in the realm of public health, exploring its potential to address public health challenges and enhance community well-being.	Develop and implement telehealth initiatives that effectively address public health challenges and contribute to enhanced community well-being.

Examine the functions and contributions of HINs in facilitating seamless communication and information exchange among health care entities for improved patient care coordination.	Enhance patient care coordination and outcomes through the effective use of HINs for seamless communication and information exchange among health care entities.
Investigate the various models and applications of telehealth, emphasizing their potential to transform health care delivery and improve patient access to medical services.	Identify and implement telehealth models and applications that significantly transform health care delivery and increase patient access to medical services.
Empower cross-state telehealth by scrutinizing licensure requirements related to telehealth, assessing their implications on health care professionals, and exploring potential enhancements to facilitate telehealth adoption through compact and multistate licenses.	Propose and advocate for changes in licensure requirements to remove barriers and facilitate wider adoption of telehealth practices among health care professionals.
Explore the role of telehealth in triage processes on hotlines, evaluating its effectiveness in efficiently directing patients to appropriate levels of care and optimizing health care resources.	Implement telehealth-based triage processes on hotlines that effectively direct patients to the appropriate level of care, thereby optimizing health care resources and reducing unnecessary in-person visits.
Analyze existing regulations governing telehealth practices to identify challenges and opportunities for improvement, ensuring a secure and effective telehealth environment while safeguarding the integrity of digital health systems.	Recommend regulatory changes to overcome existing challenges and seize opportunities for improvement, ensuring a secure, effective, and compliant telehealth practice environment.

Key Terms

Directions: Before reading, please look at this list of key terms which will he used in this chapter. If any term is unfamiliar, please see the glossary at the end of the book.

breach
enabling
health
health care
health care organizations
health care services
information
legal
mobile
networks
organizations
regulatory considerations
role
security
telehealth

A Historical Perspective

Analyzing the Evolution of Telehealth from the 1950s to Pioneering Advances in the 1960s and Beyond

On a voyage through the progression of telehealth from decades past, our investigation first makes port at the 1950s and 1960s, an era when radiographic images were wirelessly passed over voice lines, laying the foundation for what we currently regard as remote clinical care. This early application laid the foundation for broader telehealth concepts that emerged over time.

In the 1960s, through his pioneering efforts, Dr. Albert J. Sanders advanced the field significantly. Sanders marked a significant stride forward. He conducted groundbreaking experiments, utilizing closed-circuit television to provide health care services remotely, pushing the boundaries of traditional health care delivery.

Fast forwarding to 1993, it was then that the American Telemedicine Association (ATA), was formally established. This pivotal organization has been instrumental in shaping the landscape of telehealth, offering resources, setting standards, and advocating for the field. Through its efforts, ATA has emerged as a pivotal catalyst propelling the incorporation of technological solutions into improving health care outcomes. Through fostering collaboration among professionals and establishing a forum for sharing ideas and innovations within telemedicine, this organization's impact has expanded beyond merely advocating for its cause to actively cultivating progress across the entire domain. The establishment of the ATA stands out as a testament to the recognition of the potential and importance of telemedicine. Its contributions have reverberated through the years, contributing to the growth, acceptance, and continuous evolution of telehealth practices worldwide.

As technology advanced, the scope of telehealth broadened beyond traditional telemedicine. Researchers, health care professionals, and telehealth organizations have actively contributed to expanding its definitions, encompassing a wide range of services beyond remote clinical care.

Governmental bodies and health policy organizations have not remained on the sidelines. Their involvement in telehealth includes establishing guidelines, regulations, and reimbursement policies that influence its implementation and growth. Their multifaceted efforts have substantially molded the ever-evolving terrain of telehealth through meaningful involvement at various stages of development.

In this dynamic journey, the ever-evolving nature of telehealth definitions becomes evident. Ongoing technological progress, evolving approaches to health care, and shared insights among practitioners have continuously reshaped and refined our perspective on remote care delivery over time.

Charting the Course

Navigating the Transformative Landscape of Telehealth and HINs

The collaborative efforts of individuals, researchers, clinicians, and organizations have collectively contributed to the intricate tapestry that is the evolving landscape of telehealth. This transformative journey navigates through the intricate web of health information networks (HINs), recognizing their pivotal role in shaping the future of health care delivery.

Let's delve into the dynamic realm of telehealth. In this exploration, we'll uncover numerous applications that significantly impact access to quality care, enhance overall accessibility, and increase affordability. The potential for positive change in health care accessibility and quality become unmistakably clear. However, achieving these improvements requires thoughtful adjustments to the regulatory landscape.

As we navigate the latest facets of licensure, triage on hotlines, and regulatory considerations surrounding telehealth, a holistic understanding of this transformative field emerges. Comprehending these nuances empowers us to artfully guide others through telehealth's complexities, enabling them to fulfill a crucial role in making well-informed health care decisions. Our exploration focuses on three interconnected themes: telehealth, mobile health, and HINs. This journey ensures a high level of clarity with seamless transitions, allowing us to navigate the dynamic landscape of telehealth with precision and insight.

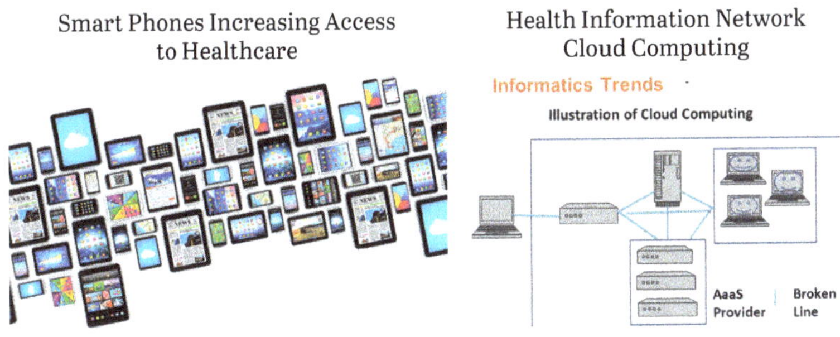

FIGURE 7.2 Mobile health technology and network.

As we venture into the dynamic realm of health informatics, consider our academic pursuit as more than a mere acquisition of knowledge—it's a strategic move toward becoming a catalyst for transformative change in health care information management. Within the intricacies of telehealth, mobile health, and HINs, we're not just exploring theoretical constructs; we're delving into the nuanced intricacies that can reshape the very foundation of health care data systems.

In the chapters ahead, we'll scrutinize the specific advantages and challenges tied to integrating telehealth and mobile health services within the health informatics landscape. Our exploration will transcend the surface, dissecting various classifications of these services, each meticulously tailored to address the diverse needs of specific patient demographics and complex health care scenarios. This chapter aims to shed light on the indispensable role of HINs, acting as the linchpin for seamless data exchange among health care entities and, consequently, elevating the efficacy of health informatics in patient care.

Empowering Cross-State Telehealth

The Importance of Compact and Multistate Licenses

In the realm of telehealth, licensed professionals are increasingly finding opportunities to extend their care across state borders. This expansion, however, requires a critical component in their professional toolkit: a compact or multistate license. A compact or multistate license empowers health care providers to seamlessly offer their services to clients situated in different states. This not only broadens the reach of their expertise, but also aligns with the evolving landscape of telehealth, in which geographical boundaries are becoming less restrictive.

This imperative is especially relevant for graduate-level students aspiring to excel in the field of telehealth. As you embark on your professional journey, acquiring a compact or multistate license becomes a strategic move, affording you the flexibility to cater to the needs of clients beyond your immediate location. Consider this license as a key that unlocks doors to a broader client base and enhances your capacity to contribute meaningfully to the dynamic and expanding field of telehealth. It is an investment in your professional versatility, positioning you to navigate the intricacies of telehealth with agility and ensuring you can make a significant impact on the accessibility and quality of health care across state lines. As graduate students in health informatics, you're not just observers; you're active contributors to the ongoing evolution of HCIS. Let's dive into this intellectually enriching journey together, armed with the analytical depth and specialized knowledge characteristic of graduate-level engagement in health informatics.

Unlocking the Potential of Telehealth

An Exploration of Virtual Health Care Services

Telehealth refers to the use of electronic information and communication technologies to support and promote long-distance clinical health care, patient and professional health-related education, public health, and health administration. The term *telehealth* is a comprehensive and evolving concept that encompasses a variety of health care services and activities delivered remotely, utilizing digital communication tools. This broad umbrella term extends across multiple dimensions, each contributing to the advancement of health care in distinct ways.

Dr. Pemberton speaks virtually to the participants in the telehealth program

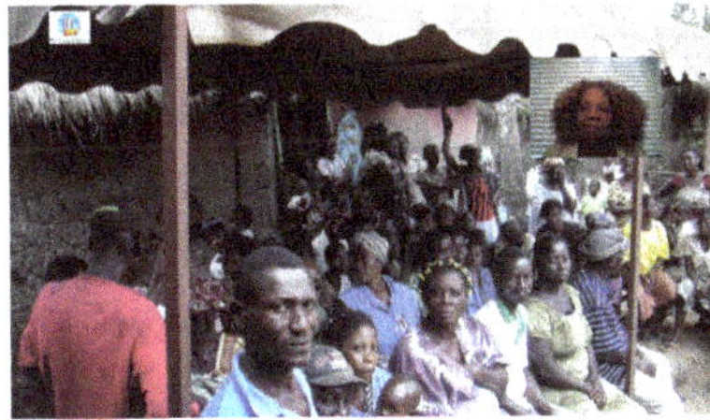

Prepare patient for evaluation by the physician in the office through a virtual computer setup

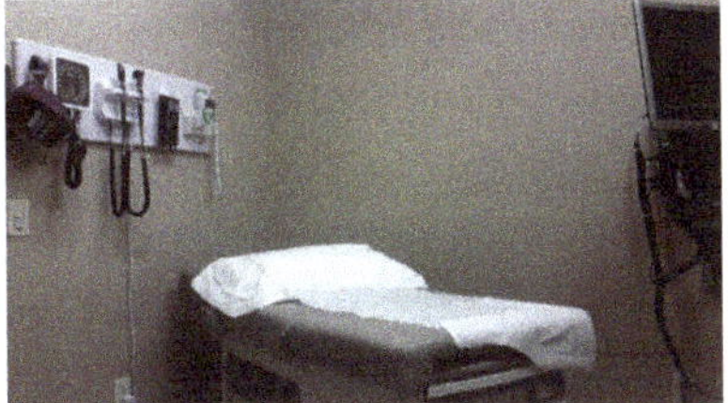

FIGURE 7.3 Telehealth in action.

From an alternative viewpoint, the provision of clinical telehealth comprises conveying medical care, examinations, diagnoses, and therapeutic game plans through advanced digital technologies like videoconferencing and long-distance checking, which allows services to be supplied remotely. This application serves to bridge geographical gaps, connecting health care providers with patients who may be at a distance.

Telehealth also plays a crucial role in health education. Digital platforms have afforded an expansive dissemination of health-related data, prospects for instruction, and educational materials to a diverse assortment of crowds, such as pupils and experts as well as participants of the overall public, via their implementation.

Additionally, telehealth now facilitates remote patient monitoring, allowing health care providers the ability to concurrently observe and administer patients' health information in real time. Through its preemptive nature, this approach enables timely interventions and customized care plans crafted to each person's distinct requirements. As health informatics graduate students, you find yourself amid a plethora of advanced technological tools, presenting abundant opportunities to conceive and implement initiatives that address the distinctive needs and challenges within the realm of health care. The landscape is rich with potential, offering a dynamic environment for the development of innovative solutions. Embrace this academic adventure as you navigate the complex intersection of health care and information technology with a keen sense of purpose and enthusiasm.

On the administrative front, telehealth involves EHR management, online appointment scheduling, and facilitating communication among health care professionals. By streamlining administrative processes and fostering collaborative decision-making in patient care, this approach not only expedites workflows, but also promotes cooperative determination in treatment options. Additionally, telehealth contributes to public health initiatives, such as disease surveillance and monitoring.

Within the domain of mental health, telehealth has proven itself a resourceful instrument capable of broadening access in impactful ways at a time when remote care has never been more essential. By enabling counseling, therapy, and assistance for those facing mental or behavioral health problems to occur from afar, this expands important psychological care to more individuals.

Ultimately, telehealth is a pivotal component of the broader digital transformation in health care. By harnessing innovations such as videoconferencing, mobile applications, wearable technologies, and additional digital means, telehealth holds the promise to substantially broaden access to care, notably better patient outcomes and elevating the overall efficiency of the health care framework. These diverse definitions collectively underscore how telehealth is employed to elevate health care delivery, education, and administration through the strategic integration of technology.

Securing Health Care Systems

Safeguarding the Heartbeat of Digital Health

As health informatics graduate students, let's immerse ourselves in the profound realm of securing health care systems, in which our role resembles that of caretakers ensuring the heartbeat of digital health remains steady and strong. Picture the principles of digital security—confidentiality, integrity, and availability—as the lifeblood coursing through the veins of our informatics journey.

Our first best practice involves defending against cyberthreats—a digital immune system, if you will. Imagine fortifying health care systems against relentless attacks, safeguarding them from the ever-present risks of cyberattacks, database breaches, and ransomware. It's akin to constructing a digital fortress, ensuring the safety of the sensitive patient data we've been entrusted with.

Now, consider the role we, as future cybersecurity professionals, play. Think of us as sentinels, standing guard over the vast realms of patient information. Our dedication goes beyond thwarting breaches; it instills confidence that patients' health data is secure. We are the stewards of digital trust, ensuring a sense of security in an increasingly interconnected health care landscape.

Transitioning to our third facet, envision firewalls and antivirus applications as the vigilant gatekeepers of the health care fortress. These tools act like security details, scrutinizing every digital visitor to ensure they are allies, not adversaries. It's an essential layer of defense, reminiscent of a security detail guaranteeing that only authorized personnel access the premises.

Navigating the Legal and Ethical Waters of Digital Security

As we shift focus to the legal and regulatory side, let's view this domain as the ethical rulebook guiding our actions in much the same way that medical ethics govern clinical practice. The legal and regulatory frameworks, including the prominent HIPAA, serve as our ethical compass in the vast sea of digital health care. These frameworks are not merely checkboxes to tick but represent a commitment to upholding patient privacy and trust—a digital Hippocratic Oath, if you will. Understanding and adhering to laws such as HIPAA become integral aspects of the oath we take as guardians of digital well-being.

Securing Health Care Systems

Best Practices and Legal Frameworks

Practices for Security in Health Care Systems

Cyberattacks, database breaches, and ransomware pose significant threats to digital security in health care. Key principles, including confidentiality, integrity, and availability, drive the need for robust security measures. Three best practices include the use of firewalls and antivirus applications, emphasizing the role of cybersecurity professionals in protecting health care organizations. This extends to the importance of employee training, awareness, and maintaining digital security. Strategies for promoting a culture of security within an organization are vital.

Legal and Regulatory Frameworks in Digital Security

When exploring the legal and regulatory landscape in digital security, specific attention is given to frameworks applicable to health care, including HIPAA and relevant laws and guidelines. This understanding is critical for maintaining compliance and safeguarding sensitive health care information.

Telehealth

Integrating Security and Privacy

In the realm of telehealth, security and privacy take center stage. Informatics students, as integral contributors, implement robust security protocols and ensure compliance with privacy regulations. Their role extends to innovating and integrating telehealth solutions with existing HCIS, creating a unified narrative in patient health management.

Real-Time Monitoring and Analytics in Telehealth

Informatics students contribute significantly to telehealth through real-time monitoring and analytics capabilities. Their involvement includes developing systems for continuous monitoring of patient health data and designing algorithms and analytics tools. This empowers health care providers to make informed decisions based on a continuous stream of remote patient data.

Navigating Policy Development and Governance in Telehealth

For graduate informatics students entering the dynamic field of telehealth, the journey involves more than technical skills. Beyond coding and system analysis, students navigate the complex terrain of policy development and governance. Crafting policies and shaping governance frameworks become essential for the seamless integration of telehealth. Challenges extend beyond lines of code, encompassing regulatory intricacies, ethical considerations, and advocating for telehealth adoption across institutional and governmental echelons.

Restoring Trust in the Aftermath of Security Breaches

Now let's navigate the aftermath of a security breach—a scenario akin to bedside manner in the digital health care realm. Security incidents disrupt not only operations, but also erode the trust patients place in the health care system. Imagine it as a breach of the sacred digital doctor–patient relationship. Our response to and management of security incidents is akin to an emergency response team rushing to a patient's aid. As health informatics professionals, our role extends beyond technicalities; it involves restoring faith and rebuilding the trust that forms the cornerstone of effective health care delivery in the digital age. Envision security not merely as a technicality but as a holistic approach intricately woven into the fabric of patient care in the digital age. Our role as guardians of digital health transcends codes and algorithms; it's about ensuring the well-being and trust of those who entrust their health information to the digital realm.

Empowering Tomorrow's Health Care Architects

Shaping the Future Through Education

As you step into the world of informatics, envision yourself as a pioneer crafting the educational landscape, shaping programs and training materials that empower health care professionals to unleash the full potential of telehealth technologies. It's about fostering a culture of continuous learning, adapting to an ever-evolving landscape, and redefining the future of health care through the transformative power of informatics.

At the Crossroads

Telehealth and Informatics

At the heart of this transformative journey lies the dynamic intersection of telehealth and informatics. Positioned at the forefront, you play a significant role in developing, implementing, and refining telehealth systems. Your contributions form the building blocks of a more connected, efficient, and patient-centered health care ecosystem. Understanding the crucial role of telehealth within the broader context of informatics positions you for pivotal roles in shaping the future of health care delivery.

Office-Based Telehealth

A Beacon of Accessibility

Let's explore office-based telehealth. Envision traditional medical offices seamlessly integrating technology to facilitate a spectrum of virtual medical consultations, diagnostics, and follow-up care. From routine check-ups to specialized consultations and mental health services, office-based telehealth emerges as a beacon of accessibility, trimming travel time and costs for patients while enhancing the overall efficiency of health care delivery.

Transitioning to Practical Applications: Bridging Knowledge to Real-World Challenges

Having explored telehealth's evolution within health informatics, we now arrive at a crucial turning point. The foundation laid thus far has equipped you with an understanding of historical contexts, technological advancements, and the critical role of informatics in shaping telehealth. Now, we shift from theory to practice, focusing on real-world applications.

Through hypothetical scenarios, you will apply your knowledge and problem-solving skills to navigate telehealth challenges. These scenarios act as a bridge between foundational learning and real-world problem-solving, preparing you to critically analyze, adapt, and implement informatics-driven solutions in evolving health care settings.

Telehealth and Informatics: Catalysts of Transformation

The intersection of telehealth and informatics is reshaping health care, offering innovative solutions to improve patient access and care delivery. As informatics students, you play a vital role in advancing telehealth systems, ensuring they are efficient, user-friendly, and capable of meeting evolving health care needs. Your contributions are instrumental in creating a more connected and patient-centered future.

Virtual Doctor Visits: Addressing Health Care Challenges

The COVID-19 pandemic underscored the necessity of virtual health care solutions, particularly for vulnerable populations such as cancer patients. Visiting health care facilities posed significant risks, making access to essential care more challenging. In response, virtual doctor visits became a critical solution. Patients could attend appointments from a clinical setting while their doctors assessed and discussed treatment plans via video.

A Virtual Lifeline for Cancer Patients

This approach not only ensured continuity of care but also provided a safer alternative for patients to consult with their doctors without unnecessary exposure to risks. Even when patients were physically present in a clinical setting, the doctor's remote participation classified these encounters as telehealth. The defining aspect of telehealth lies in its ability to bridge geographical barriers and enhance accessibility through technology.

Innovation in Patient Care

Integrating virtual consultations into health care workflows has proven invaluable, not just as a response to emergencies but as a long-term solution for improving patient-provider interactions. These advancements exemplify how health informatics enhances care delivery, making health services more adaptable, efficient, and patient-focused.

One cannot help but acknowledge the unforeseen impact this iniative had. In hindsight, had there been the foresight to anticipate the remarkable sequence of revelations, mental preparation for the subsequent exposures would have been more prudent.

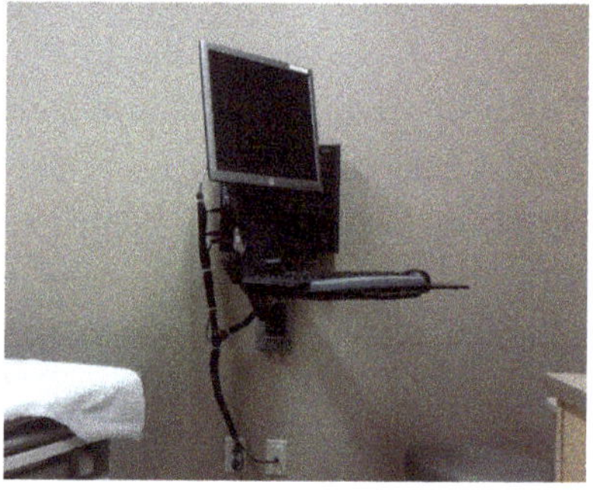

FIGURE 7.4 Virtual health care.

A Constant Presence in the Face of Challenges

Throughout this transformative process, the integration of health informatics played a critical role in improving patient care. A dedicated nurse was present to provide ongoing support; ensuring patients received timely assistance when needed. This transformation involved leveraging technology to enhance communication, streamline workflows, and improve decision-making. As a result, even amid unforeseen challenges, the health care team was able to maintain high-quality care. This achievement underscores the vital role of technology in revolutionizing health care practices and shaping the future of patient care.

Through the camera feed, the physician would engage the patient in dialogue, requesting they indicate any regions that elicited concern. Had I possessed the foresight to foresee the extraordinary sequence of revelations that teetered on the cusp of origination, I would have endeavored to steel myself in a frame of mind more befitting to welcome without the unforeseen exposures that later emerged from the shadows. A nurse was always there, ready to help.

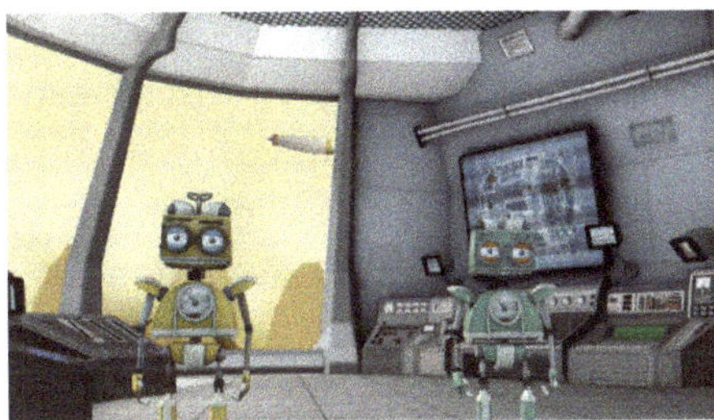
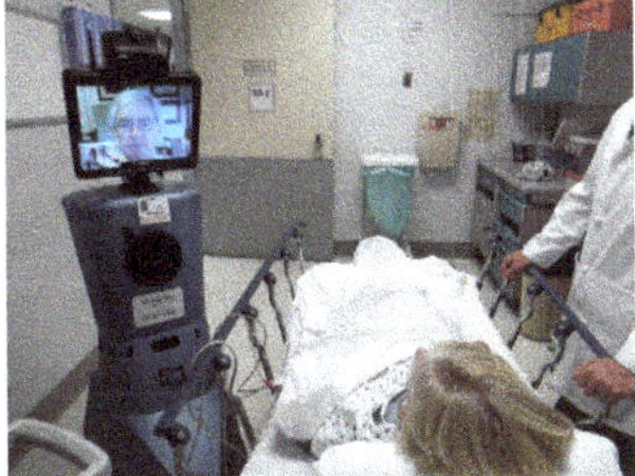

FIGURE 7.5 Robotics.

Revolutionizing Patient Care

A Glimpse Into Technological Advancements

Let's dive into the fascinating realm of patient monitoring through technology, a concept akin to experiencing a highly advanced phone call. Believe it or not, patients genuinely appreciate it! In 2004, Cisco, a technology giant, experimented with a robot doctor designed to visit patients in the hospital. Yes, you heard that right—a robot doctor! During this intriguing experiment, even the esteemed Barbara Bush, the former first lady, actively participated in the demonstration. To her delight, she found the constant availability and unwavering dedication of the robotic physician truly remarkable. It created a sense that the doctor was virtually omnipresent, always there to address her needs, regardless of the hour.

Fast forward to today, and we witness the evolution of telehealth as a powerful tool, allowing patients to conveniently access high-quality medical care from the comfort of their own spaces. Yet, as we embrace these advancements, it's crucial to acknowledge that the potential of telehealth goes beyond convenience. There's a pressing need for further development and study to explore its ability to enhance outcomes, especially for those who lack nearby specialist access. The journey of technology in health care is a continuous exploration, offering not only convenience but also the promise of broader and more inclusive health care solutions for everyone.

Challenges of Office-Based Telehealth

Challenges, however, accompany the benefits of office-based telehealth. Connectivity issues, data security concerns, and the need for specialized training for health care professionals engaging in telehealth are notable hurdles. Navigating these challenges is imperative for the seamless integration of office-based telehealth into mainstream health care practices. To comprehend this domain, key terms and concepts such as telemedicine, virtual consultations, and EHRs become foundational. Understanding these concepts is essential for students to navigate the nuances of office-based telehealth and its integration into contemporary health care systems.

Homecare and Public Telehealth

Shifting focus to homecare telehealth, this variant extends health care services beyond clinical settings, bringing medical expertise into the comfort of patients' homes. By emphasizing the use of technology to monitor, diagnose, and treat patients remotely, homecare telehealth utilizes mobile health applications for real-time communication and access to health information.

In the realm of public health, telehealth initiatives take center stage, extending health care reach to broader populations and emphasizing preventive measures. Public telehealth programs

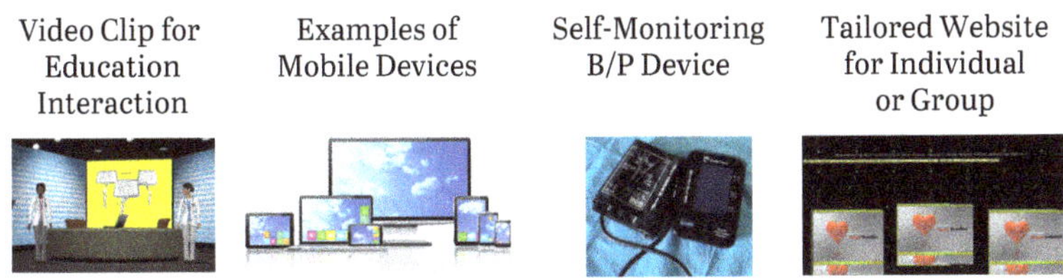

FIGURE 7.6 Meaningful use of mobile technology.

leverage technology to address public health challenges and improve overall community well-being. Examples of such programs, from vaccination campaigns to real-time monitoring of public health indicators, illustrate the practical applications of telehealth in addressing public health challenges.

Unveiling the Power of HINs in Telehealth

As you step into the realm of telehealth, consider the pivotal role played by HINs. Picture these networks as the backbone, orchestrating the seamless exchange of health information in the telehealth landscape. Envision HINs transforming the telehealth system into an integrated and collaborative network.

Navigating the Vast Terrain of Telehealth Approaches

Transition smoothly to various telehealth approaches and imagine yourself navigating through a diverse array of tools and methodologies. From store-and-forward models to real-time video consultations, dive into the spectrum of telehealth. Each approach has its unique strengths, and your critical evaluation skills will be key.

Mastering the Language of Telehealth Strategies

Enter the world of telehealth strategies with key terms like *synchronous* and *asynchronous telehealth*, *remote patient monitoring*, and *teletriage*. This linguistic foundation sets the stage for your comparative analysis so that you can weigh the strengths and weaknesses of different telehealth approaches. Keep in mind, HINs play a crucial role in creating a cohesive and integrated telehealth landscape.

Equipping Yourself for Impactful Contributions in Telehealth

Navigate through interconnected dimensions and picture yourself equipped with the knowledge and skills needed to contribute meaningfully to the evolving field of telehealth. Whether it's office-based, homecare, or public health telehealth, you're gaining a nuanced understanding—from foundational concepts to practical illustrations.

Decoding the Legal Landscape of Telehealth Licensure

Delve into the intricate landscape of telehealth with an understanding of its legal implications. Licensure is a cornerstone shaping the regulatory framework to ensure ethical and lawful health care services in remote environments. It's not just a formality; it establishes trust between practitioners and patients.

Overcoming Telehealth Licensure Challenges

Recognize the challenges in telehealth licensure, especially the variability across jurisdictions. Your role involves advocating for standardized licensure requirements. Actively participate in discussions and initiatives aiming to create a more cohesive and uniform system. Your engagement is pivotal for the ongoing development of ethical and legally sound telehealth practices.

Embracing the Vital Role of Triage in Telehealth

For students exploring the multifaceted world of telehealth, grasp the paramount role of triage. Imagine yourself in the realm of hotlines, efficiently assessing and categorizing patients' needs for timely and appropriate care. Your involvement in hotline triage contributes to optimizing resource allocation and addressing urgent matters efficiently. This personalized journey speaks to your expertise as a graduate-level health informatics student, emphasizing the significance of each step in your exploration of telehealth.

Summary

In conclusion, as we wrap up our exploration of telehealth regulation, acknowledge its fundamental role in ensuring ethical and lawful health care practices. Embrace the importance of compliance and remain mindful of the challenges that shape the telehealth landscape. Your awareness and engagement in this aspect positions you not just as learners, but as active contributors to the continued development of telehealth regulation. Chapter 7 illuminated the complexities and critical aspects of hotline triage and telehealth regulation, offering you a holistic perspective as you journey through the multifaceted world of telehealth and informatics. The regulatory landscape is viewed as a guide governing telehealth practices. By analyzing existing regulations, identifying challenges, and envisioning opportunities for improvement, a vision of a secure and effective telehealth environment emerges. As you move forward, carry this understanding with you. You're not just students; you are contributors shaping the future of telehealth. Your journey is more than a study—it's a meaningful exploration into a field that depends on your insights and engagement. Embrace your role, and let your contribution be a beacon in the ever-evolving landscape of telehealth and informatics.

Chapter Review Questions

Directions: Consider what you learned in this chapter as you respond to the health care scenario and questions.

Health Care Scenario: Exploring the Possibilities of Telehealth

Dr. Alice Brown is a health care administrator in a rural community hospital. The hospital has recently received a grant to implement a comprehensive telehealth program aimed at improving access to health care for residents who live in remote areas. The telehealth program includes telemedicine services, mobile health applications, and the development of a HIN to connect various health care providers in the region.

As part of the implementation process, Dr. Brown is tasked with ensuring the program meets clinical, educational, and community care needs. She begins by analyzing historical data on telehealth, learning about the pioneering efforts in the 1950s and 1960s, and how organizations like the ATA have shaped the field. Dr. Brown also reviews current regulations and reimbursement policies to ensure compliance and sustainability of the telehealth services.

Dr. Brown collaborates with clinicians, IT professionals, and policymakers to address the challenges of implementing telehealth technologies. She focuses on ensuring the program is user-friendly for both health care providers and patients. Additionally, Dr. Brown emphasizes the importance of critical thinking and problem solving among her team to adapt telehealth solutions to the specific needs of the community.

The hospital plans to launch the telehealth program with several key services: virtual consultations for chronic disease management, remote monitoring of patients with mobile health devices, educational webinars for health care professionals on the latest telehealth practices, and a HIN to facilitate data sharing among health care providers.

Multiple Choice Questions

1. What was one of the earliest applications of telehealth in the 1950s and 1960s?
   a. Videoconferencing for mental health therapy
   b. Remote surgery using robotic technology
   c. Wireless transmission of radiographic images
   d. Telehealth applications for homecare
2. Which organization, established in 1993, has been pivotal in shaping the landscape of telehealth?
   a. World Health Organization (WHO)
   b. Centers for Disease Control and Prevention (CDC)
   c. American Telemedicine Association (ATA)
   d. National Institutes of Health (NIH)

3. What is a key benefit of telehealth highlighted in the case scenario?
   a. Increased hospital admissions
   b. Enhanced access to health care for remote residents
   c. Higher costs for health care services
   d. Reduced need for health care education
4. What role did Dr. Albert J. Sanders play in the evolution of telehealth?
   a. He invented mobile health applications.
   b. He established the ATA.
   c. He conducted experiments with closed-circuit television for remote health care.
   d. He developed telehealth policies and regulations.
5. Which of the following is *not* a component of Dr. Brown's telehealth program?
   a. Virtual consultations for chronic disease management
   b. In-person health fairs for community engagement
   c. Remote monitoring of patients with mobile health devices
   d. Educational webinars for health care professionals
6. How does the ATA contribute to the field of telehealth?
   a. By providing direct health care services to patients
   b. By setting standards, offering resources, and advocating for telehealth
   c. By developing telehealth technologies
   d. By training health care professionals in traditional medicine
7. What is one of the challenges Dr. Brown faces in implementing the telehealth program?
   a. Ensuring the program is user-friendly for both health care providers and patients
   b. Reducing the number of health care professionals in the hospital

   c. Limiting the types of health care services offered
   d. Increasing the cost of health care services

8. Why is critical thinking emphasized in Dr. Brown's approach to telehealth implementation?

   a. To reduce the need for technological advancements
   b. To adapt telehealth solutions to the specific needs of the community
   c. To limit the use of telehealth technologies
   d. To increase the complexity of health care service

Answer Key

1. (c) Wireless transmission of radiographic images
2. (c) American Telemedicine Association (ATA)
3. (b) Enhanced access to health care for remote residents
4. (c) He conducted experiments with closed-circuit television for remote health care.
5. (b) In-person health fairs for community engagement
6. (b) By setting standards, offering resources, and advocating for telehealth
7. (a) Ensuring the program is user-friendly for both health care providers and patients
8. (b) To adapt telehealth solutions to the specific needs of the community

Recommended Reading

Board on Health Care Services & Institute of Medicine. (2012). *The role of telehealth in an evolving health care environment: Workshop summary.* The National Academies Press. https://www.ncbi.nlm.nih.gov/books/NBK207151/

Joshi, A. U., & Welsh, B. M. (2023, December 12). How large healthcare providers use telehealth and telemedicine. *Forbes*. https://www.

forbes.com/sites/forbesbooksauthors/2023/12/12/how-large-health care-providers-use-telehealth-and-telemedicine/

McElroy, J. A., Day, T. M., & Becevic, M. (2020). The influence of telehealth for better health across communities. *Preventing Chronic Disease*, *17*, E64. https://doi.org/10.5888/pcd17.200254

Patel, N. G. (2023, December 15). Unlocking healthcare trends and considerations for investors. *Forbes*. https://www.forbes.com/sites/forbesbusinesscouncil/2023/12/15/unlocking-healthcare-trends-and-considerations-for-investors/

Figure Credits

Fig. 7.1a: Copyright © 2010 Depositphotos/Alekcey.

Fig. 7.1b: Copyright © 2013 by Intel Free Press (CC BY-SA 4.0) at https://commons.wikimedia.org/wiki/File:Suitable_Technologies_Beam_telepresence_robot.jpg.

Fig. 7.1c: Copyright © 2012 Depositphotos/Amnez.

Fig. 7.1d: Copyright © 2014 Depositphotos/macrovector.

Fig. 7.1e: Copyright © 2019 Depositphotos/MarySan_.

Fig. 7.1f: Copyright © 2012 Depositphotos/jamesgroup.

Fig. 7.2a: Copyright © 2015 Depositphotos/scanrail.

Fig. 7.3a: Copyright © 2021 by Freida Pemberton (CC BY 4.0) at https://crimsonpublishers.com/cojnh/pdf/COJNH.000665.pdf.

Fig. 7.5a: Generated using Nawmal. Copyright © by Technologies Nawmal, Inc. Reprinted with permission.

Fig. 7.5b: Copyright © 2015 by Jill Braden Balderas (CC BY-ND 4.0) at https://www.northcarolinahealthnews.org/2015/07/02/13236/.

Fig. 7.6a: Generated using Nawmal. Copyright © by Technologies Nawmal, Inc. Reprinted with permission.

Fig. 7.6b: Copyright © 2014 Depositphotos/fkdkondmi.

Chapter 8

Digital Security to Protect Sensitive Patient Data and Other Health Care Information

Introduction

Chapter 8 invites us into the critical realm of digital security. This chapter emphasizes the paramount importance of safeguarding individual medical records and explores the intricate challenges faced by medical institutions in the ever-evolving digital landscape.

The purpose of this chapter is to empower graduate health informatics students with the essential knowledge and skills needed to navigate and secure the digital health care landscape. By understanding regulatory frameworks, historical transitions, and real-world vulnerabilities, students will learn to develop and implement robust security measures, ensuring the integrity and privacy of sensitive patient data. This chapter aims to transform students into proactive guardians of health care information, equipped to handle the challenges of a digitalized health care environment.

Chapter 8 is significant as it addresses the critical need for enhanced digital security in the transition from paper to EHRs. This shift brings heightened security concerns that require informed and strategic responses. By examining real-world breaches, identifying vulnerabilities, and evaluating preventive measures, this chapter highlights the necessity of strong digital security protocols in health care.

As you are immersed in the complexities of digital security within health care, you will uncover the intricate challenges faced by medical institutions and address the inherent threats and nuances of this dynamic environment. This exploration goes beyond defensive measures, inviting you to navigate the spectrum from protective strategies to potential vulnerabilities. By diligently pursuing this course, you will acquire a comprehensive understanding of how to reliably safeguard the integrity and privacy of sensitive patient records.

Amid the excitement of technological progress, concerns about the security of health information are palpable. Questions linger, such as, "Can you truly trust your paper records?" This apprehension is valid, given that paper records lack the robust security features of modern digital systems.

During this transition, discussions revolve around vulnerabilities inherent in both paper and digital records. Presentations emphasize the accessibility issues with paper records and underscore the growing concerns about the security of digital health records. It is akin to upgrading from a basic padlock to a cutting-edge security system tailored for the digital landscape. The objective is to guarantee the impeccable security of health information handled by future professionals like yourselves.

As you master these complexities, you position yourself as a steward of sensitive health care data—a pivotal role in the modern health care landscape. Chapter 8 serves as the canvas for your in-depth exploration of digital security, a skill set demanded by the industry and essential for future health care information guardians.

With the defense of health care data gaining prominence, your expertise becomes crucial in shaping the trajectory of health informatics progress. May this chapter not only serve as a learning resource but also as a foundational steppingstone in your journey to becoming an essential member in the constantly evolving domain of electronic safeguarding within health care.

Objectives That Lead to Outcomes

Specific objectives and their corresponding expected outcomes for this chapter are outlined. The following table aligns key objectives with their outcomes, providing a clear and detailed understanding of what learners should achieve and comprehend upon completion. These objectives will guide the planning and execution of the HIS project, ensuring it aligns with the organization's strategic goals and principles of effective project management and organizational management.

Objective	Outcome
Identify and analyze common cyberattacks in health care and evaluate preventive measures and response strategies.	Create a detailed report documenting common cyber-attacks in health care, assessing current preventive measures and response strategies, and proposing improvements.
Investigate real-world breaches and vulnerabilities in health care databases and propose strategies to enhance database security.	Develop a case study compilation of real-world health care data breaches, identify key vulnerabilities, and present actionable strategies for enhancing database security.
Explore ethical considerations in health data integrity and develop best practices for maintaining data accuracy and reliability.	Produce guidelines that address ethical considerations in health data integrity and establish best practices for ensuring data accuracy and reliability in health care systems.
Evaluate existing security frameworks (e.g., HIPAA) in health care and formulate recommendations for framework implementation and improvement.	Conduct a comprehensive analysis of current security frameworks, such as HIPAA, and develop a set of recommendations for effective implementation and potential improvements.
Understand the life cycle of health information and related legal/ethical principles and assess health informatics roles in ensuring information accuracy and confidentiality.	Create a life cycle model of health information, highlighting legal and ethical principles, and assess the roles of health informatics professionals in maintaining information accuracy and confidentiality.

Analyze technological impacts on health care delivery and develop strategies to adapt health informatics systems to evolving health care models.	Generate a strategic plan that analyzes the impact of emerging technologies in health care delivery and outlines adaptive strategies for health informatics systems to align with evolving health care models.

Key Terms

Directions: Before reading, please look at this list of key terms that will be used in this chapter. If any term is unfamiliar, please see the glossary at the end of the book.

database breaches
health care delivery system
health information
integrity issues
security protection frameworks
security systems

Evolution of Digital Health Records and Security Measures

The evolution of health records and security measures has undergone significant transformation over time. Before the 1900s, medical documentation was primarily paper-based, with records manually written and stored in physical archives. Security measures were rudimentary, relying on locked cabinets and physical safeguards. With the advent of the early digital era (1980s–1999), health care institutions began transitioning to basic EHR systems, though digital security remained limited. The 2000s–2023 saw a rapid expansion in health IT, with widespread adoption of EHRs, cloud storage, multifactor authentication, and stricter privacy regulations to protect patient data (Okpara-Oguadimma, 2024). Moving forward, from 2024 and beyond, the integration of AI, blockchain encryption, and real-time interoperability is expected to further enhance data security and accessibility, leading to a more interconnected and patient-centric health care ecosystem.

The following table outlines key milestones in the development of digital health records and security measures, highlighting their evolution from paper-based systems to AI-driven advancements.

TABLE 8.1 Timeline of the Advancement in Digital Health Records and Protective Security

Aspect	Emergence of Health Records (Pre–1900s)	Early Digital Era (1980s–1999)	Recent Advancements (2000s–2023)	Future Trends (2024 & beyond)
Health Records	Paper-based records	Basic electronic systems	Wide adoption of EHRs	Interoperability and AI-driven health records
Security Measures	Physical safeguards (locks, keys)	Limited digital security	Introduction of encryption and access controls	Blockchain and advanced encryption
Data Accessibility	Localized, manual retrieval	Limited remote access	Web-based systems and cloud storage	Mobile access and real-time updates
Interoperability	Minimal data exchange	Limited data sharing	Push for interoperability standards	Seamless data exchange across systems
User Authentication	Signature based	Basic username/ password	Multifactor authentication	Biometric and adaptive authentication
Privacy Compliance	Informal, ethical guidelines	Emerging regulatory frameworks	Stricter compliance regulations	Global standards and data governance
Data Breach Response	Manual detection and response	Reactive measures	Proactive monitoring and incident response	AI-driven threat detection and response
Integration with IoT	Nonexistent	Initial integration with devices	Extensive connectivity with IoT devices	AI-powered analytics for IoT data
Patient Involvement	Limited access to records	Patient portals introduced	Patient-controlled data sharing	Increased patient engagement

Securing Patient Data

Navigating Vulnerabilities in Paper-Based Records

Your expertise holds immense significance in shaping the trajectory of health informatics progress. Let's explore the historical context of patient record security, predating the current digital era. In the era before EHRs, health care heavily relied on paper-based records, and security concerns were a constant presence.

During those times, vulnerabilities arose from the use of paper records. The physical accessibility of patient information in open medical facilities created tangible risks. Imagine the easily reachable environments where paper records were stored, often within arm's length. The simplicity with which individuals could access and potentially misuse information raised significant concerns.

Adding to the vulnerability was the absence of a systematic audit trail. Unlike today's digital systems that meticulously log every access instance, paper records lacked the ability to track who accessed them, when, and for what purpose. This lack of accountability meant breaches could occur undetected. Moreover, human error, an inherent element in any system, was more pronounced in a paper-based environment. Misplacement or misfiling could lead to the wrong person gaining access to sensitive patient records. Inefficient communication and information sharing among health care providers or institutions further heightened the risks.

To illustrate the potential harm, consider a scenario when a misplaced paper record results in the wrong person gaining access to a patient's sensitive health information. The lack of a clear audit trail means that such a breach could go unnoticed for a significant period, compromising patient privacy and confidentiality. Your role as a health informatics professional is pivotal in addressing and mitigating these historical challenges. By understanding the vulnerabilities of the past, you are better equipped to contribute to the ongoing advancement of secure and efficient HCIS.

Charting the Security Shift

Transitioning From Paper to Digital Health Records

The shift from paper to digital health records strategically addressed vulnerabilities, introducing encryption, robust access controls, audit trails, secure authentication, and authorization methods. This evolution aimed to mitigate vulnerabilities prevalent in the analog era. EHRs brought forth encryption as a shield, ensuring patient information remained secure. Robust access controls acted as gatekeepers, permitting entry only to those with legitimate reasons.

Audit trails emerged as meticulous recordkeepers, enhancing accountability and enabling swift rectification of breaches. Authentication methods, absent in the paper-based realm, became the first line of defense in the digital frontier, ensuring only authorized personnel accessed patient data. While progress has strengthened digital defenses, ongoing prudence is essential. The dynamic digital landscape presents new challenges, demanding our continuous attunement to technology's pulse. Our role in health care information management requires anticipating and addressing potential pitfalls proactively.

Historical concerns about patient record security serve as cautionary tales, urging a proactive stance. In health informatics, let's not view security measures as checkboxes but as integral components of our ethical responsibility. Lessons from the past underscore the need for a holistic approach, combining technological prowess with ethical considerations. Despite digital challenges, historical concerns about patient record security have evolved.

Our journey in health informatics involves navigating present complexities while appreciating historical context. The transition from paper to digital responds to longstanding concerns about patient information security. As stewards of health data, let's explore these historical intricacies, recognizing the lessons they offer for our evolving role in health care information management.

Ushering in HIPAA

Safeguarding Health Information on a Legislative Canvas

As health informatics graduate students, let's recognize HIPAA as a foundational pillar. Rather than a mere list of directives, it constitutes a dedication to safeguarding privacy, maintaining security, and handling information responsibly—an abiding principle that must continue to guide us as our domain constantly changes.

In 1996, responding to societal concerns, the U.S. Congress enacted HIPAA, a legislative giant rooted in the sanctity of health records. Its multifaceted objectives unfold through the Privacy Rule, establishing national standards that grant patients unprecedented control over their medical records and personal health information as in patient portals. This shift marks a pivotal moment in the information privacy landscape.

Another guardian within HIPAA, the Security Rule, intensifies the focus on protecting electronic protected health information. Stringent standards uphold confidentiality, integrity, and availability—addressing the digital age's need for robust security protocols.

Simultaneously, the Transactions and Code Sets Rule acts as a harmonizing force, standardizing electronic exchanges of health care data for enhanced efficiency and security within the intricate health care ecosystem. The Unique Identifiers Rule, akin to a digital nomenclature, assigns distinct markers to health care entities, ensuring smooth electronic transactions and minimizing friction in the exchange of crucial health care information.

ESSENTIALS OF A NOMENCLATURE

- Developed to define characteristics of the system's purpose
- Classification of nursing intensity would consist of terms that describe patient characteristics that impact resources needed for care
- Billing nomenclature would consist of terms that describe actions and/or procedures that can be used in billing to a third party

KEY TRAITS OF AN EFFECTIVE NOMENCLATURE FOR STRUCTURED DATA

Researchers have delineated the characteristics of a "good" nomenclature for purposes of structured data capture, storage, analysis, and reporting:

- domain completeness
- granularity
- parsimony
- synonymy
- nonambiguity
- nonredundancy
- clinical utility
- multiple axes
- combinatorial

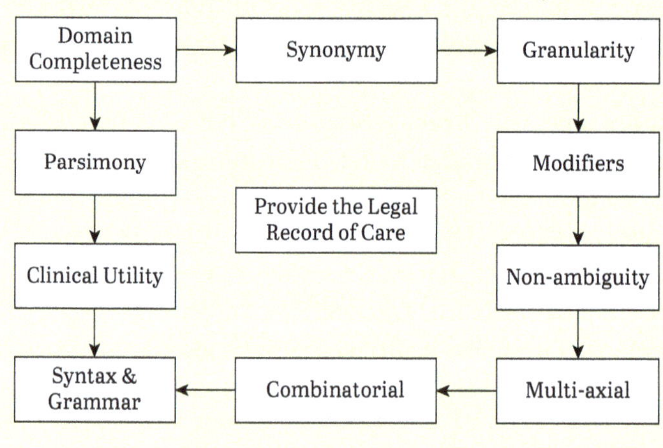

FIGURE 8.1 An excellent system.

Essentially, HIPAA orchestrates a delicate balance, navigating between the necessity for health care entities to share information for treatment and the unwavering safeguarding of patients' sensitive health data. The overarching objective is clear: Forge trust between patients and health care organizations through a stringent tapestry of guidelines and safeguards.

Beyond being a regulatory chore, compliance with HIPAA emerges as a linchpin for upholding patient trust in the health care system. Extracting valuable lessons from historical intricacies that have shaped our field, our role as health informatics professionals goes beyond navigating the complexities of the present—it involves gleaning insights that echo through the corridors of time.

Examples of Fortifying Health Care

Navigating Security Frameworks

Navigating the complex world of health informatics involves understanding contemporary security frameworks protecting patient data in our digital world. Let's explore these measures in a way that resonates with our roles as future health care leaders.

In today's interconnected world, encryption continues to act as a digital fortress around patient information. Within health care, it ensures that sensitive data in EHRs remains private and available exclusively to authorized staff.

Access controls are like diligent gatekeepers in a hospital, deciding who gets access and granting varied permission levels based on roles. This mirrors the balance between collaboration and the essential need to safeguard patient information.

Audit trails serve as silent observers, recording every patient interaction and acting as an ethical compass. In a transparent health care setting, they swiftly identify and address any deviations from standard protocol. Authentication methods have evolved into digital identity cards, ensuring only those with legitimate reasons can access patient data. Establishing trust in every digital exchange is crucial, as logging in is just the start of protecting private medical information.

As we embrace these security measures, our journey doesn't end. The dynamic digital landscape continually presents new challenges. We must be vigilant custodians, adapting our strategies to counter evolving threats. It's a continuous dialogue between technology and ethics, using the tools at our disposal to protect not just data but the trust patients place in the health care system.

Our role as health informatics professionals is about upholding the ethical fabric of health care. These security frameworks are not mere technicalities; they're pillars supporting the foundation of trust. As we navigate these platforms, let's ensure every measure implemented is a testament to our commitment to excellence and integrity in health care information management.

Our evolving role requires us to remain vigilant to technological advancements, anticipating and mitigating potential risks (Haney & Lutters, 2020). Past challenges in patient record security serve as valuable lessons, emphasizing the need for a proactive approach. This is our opportunity not just to manage information but to protect it—blending historical insights with cutting-edge innovation to ensure a future where patient data remains secure and serves as a foundation for excellence in health care.

Defending the Health Frontline

Safeguarding Against Common Cyberattacks in Health Informatics

As we advance our ever-growing reliance in health informatics on digital systems, we must sharpen our awareness of the myriad challenges, particularly in the face of cyberattacks. One prominent threat is posed by data breaches, when malicious actors target health care organizations to gain unauthorized access to sensitive patient information. This data, encompassing personal and medical records, holds significant value on illicit markets, leading to potential ramifications such as identity theft and insurance fraud.

Another formidable challenge comes in the form of ransomware attacks, a tactic employed by cybercriminals to encrypt crucial health care data. The subsequent demand for a ransom in exchange for data release can swiftly disrupt medical services, potentially compromising patient safety. Succumbing to ransom demands is not a foolproof solution and may inadvertently support further criminal activities.

The impact extends to hindering access to patient records, a cornerstone of informed decision-making in health care. In a field in which every second counts, the inability to swiftly retrieve crucial patient information can have serious consequences. Perhaps most strikingly, these disruptions can lead to a kind of chaos within the organization. Picture the intricate orchestration of health care professionals, support staff, and systems harmoniously working together to provide quality care. Now envision the disarray introduced by a sudden disruption—appointments missed, communications faltering, and a sense of disorder that challenges the very essence of our mission in health informatics.

As health informatics graduate students, this isn't just an academic exercise. Many organizations mandate that personnel undergo a series of concise certification classes to safeguard records and ensure the smooth functioning of systems, thereby mitigating the risk of potential cyberattacks.

Unveiling the Impact

Distributed Denial-of-Service Attacks as Digital Storms in Health Care

While the technical facets of distributed denial-of-service (DDoS) attacks must be acknowledged, we ought to consider too their meaningful human impact, for it is people who ultimately endure such online onslaughts. Let's delve into the impact of DDoS attacks on health care. Imagine a hospital's online systems as the beating heart of its operations, coordinating appointments, managing patient records, and facilitating seamless communication among health care professionals. Now picture a DDoS attack as an unexpected storm that hits this digital heartbeat.

A technical DDoS attack aims to overwhelm online systems by generating an excessive amount of traffic, thereby rendering the services inaccessible to valid users through volume alone. However, the human impact goes beyond the technical disruption. Consider a scenario when a hospital's scheduling system becomes inaccessible due to a DDoS attack. Appointments cannot be made or rescheduled, leading to a ripple effect on patient care. Patients might miss crucial appointments, affecting the continuity of their treatment plans. This disruption isn't just about servers and networks; it directly interferes with the timely and personalized care that individuals rely on.

Moreover, think about the health care professionals relying on real-time access to patient records during a DDoS attack. If they can't retrieve vital information promptly, decision-making may be compromised, potentially affecting patient outcomes. The human consequences extend to delays in critical diagnoses, treatment plans, and overall health care delivery.

In essence, acknowledging the meaningful human impact of DDoS attacks in health care involves understanding how these disruptions can disrupt the interconnected processes that ensure timely and effective patient care. While servers and technicalities matter, what truly counts are the people whose health and wellness rely on these systems working seamlessly.

Our efforts to enhance health care systems underscore the vital need to defend against threats to continuity and well-being, as securing such services determines the welfare of those dependent on the aims we pursue. In an effort to maintain health care continuity and ultimately shield societal wellness, we are striving to fortify systems for the delivery of medical care during this time.

Charting the Course: A Comprehensive Approach to Cybersecurity in Health Care for Health Informatics Graduates

The increasing interconnectivity of medical devices introduces vulnerabilities that cyberattackers exploit. Compromised devices can result in incorrect treatment delivery, endangering patients, and disrupting critical health care operations.

Phishing and social engineering techniques remain prevalent, with the human factor playing a crucial role in cyber risks. Deceptive emails, messages, and phone calls often trick health care staff into divulging sensitive information, compromising patient confidentiality and organizational security.

Internally, insider threats pose significant risks, whether through intentional malicious actions or unintentional negligence.

Mishandling data or facilitating external attacks can lead to breaches, unauthorized access, and reputational damage.

Supply chain vulnerabilities further complicate the cybersecurity landscape. Health care organizations, reliant on networks of vendors and suppliers, can suffer the consequences of attacks targeting third-party entities. A compromised supply chain partner may introduce malware or enable unauthorized access, exposing sensitive information.

For health informatics graduates, addressing these threats requires a multifaceted approach. Implementing robust cybersecurity measures, conducting regular security assessments, and providing comprehensive employee training are essential. By collaborating with cybersecurity specialists, applying industry-recommended safeguards, and staying informed on emerging threats, organizations can protect sensitive patient data and maintain trust in health care through a comprehensive digital defense strategy.

Strategies to Strengthen Digital Concerns and Prevent Cyber Intruders

In the ever-evolving domain of cyberspace, databases play a crucial role as secure repositories for invaluable information. These databases are fortified with advanced security measures, functioning as digital safeguards against unauthorized access and potential cyber threats.

Within these digital repositories lie the essential elements of our interconnected society: critical data, records, and information that are indispensable for various sectors such as businesses, health care, education, and more. These databases are central hubs, managing, organizing, and facilitating the retrieval of information efficiently. For graduate-level informatics students, understanding the significance of databases goes beyond their technical functionalities. Recognizing the dual role of databases as protectors and custodians underscores their pivotal position in the realm of information management, influencing the dynamics of our interconnected world.

Guardians of the Digital Realm

Fortifying Cybersecurity Through Esteemed Organizations and Threat Mitigation

In the ever-evolving landscape of cyberspace, several esteemed organizations take the lead in ensuring digital security. These prominent cyber organizations, including the Cybersecurity and Infrastructure Security Agency, International Information System Security Certification Consortium, and Electronic Frontier Foundation, each crucially contribute to shielding our digital realms through their indispensable parts. Their efforts contribute significantly to the protection of invaluable information, reinforcing the integrity of our interconnected society.

While the ITL, the commonly known Information Technology Laboratory within the National Institute of Standards and Technology (NIST), carries out foundational computer science research by exploring emerging areas, it also reinforces established work to further knowledge in this evolving field. The NIST promotes the U.S. economy and public welfare by providing technical leadership for the nation's measurement and standards infrastructure (International Cybersecurity Standardization Working Group, 2015). The ITL develops tests, test methods, reference data, proof of concept implementations, and technical analyses to advance the development and productive use of information technology.

Among the foremost threats are password pirates, adept at probing for weak points akin to attempting to decipher an intricate lock with rudimentary tools. Thus, the imperative arises to fortify the digital gates with robust and complex access codes, rendering unauthorized entry a formidable challenge. Simultaneously, the realm contends with phishing phantoms, insidious actors who assume the semblance of familiar contacts in pursuit of deceitful objectives. Navigating this landscape demands discernment and a shrewd awareness to discern genuine allies from potential adversaries donned in deceptive garb.

Ensuring our digital defenses are up-to-date is as essential as a health care professional regularly updating their skills. Just like neglecting security updates leaves vulnerabilities, overlooking ongoing education in health care can expose us to potential risks. As stewards of these digital strongholds, it behooves us to ensure the continual enhancement and fortification of our defenses.

Strategies Against Insider Threats, Encryption Safeguards, and Data Governance

In the realm of digital defense, insider intruders pose a potential threat, emphasizing the need for meticulous oversight to scrutinize trusted custodians and preempt internal compromises. Encryption algorithms serve as a secure code, making sensitive information indecipherable to unauthorized entities. The effectiveness of these safeguards depends on the delicate balance between accessibility for legitimate users and imperviousness to nefarious actors.

Inadvertent data exposure, akin to misplacing or sharing a patient's medical chart, underscores the importance of meticulous data governance to ensure that only those entrusted with the knowledge have access. As health informatics professionals, envision our role as stewards navigating the evolving health care technology landscape. Each technological advancement, like AI, telehealth, and blockchain, represents a pivotal moment, expanding our responsibilities beyond mere users to custodians.

AI offers insights with an ethical imperative, ensuring unbiased application in health care decision-making. Telehealth brings health care to fingertips, requiring navigation of accessibility and inclusivity. Blockchain, a guardian of trust, promises enhanced security, demanding careful integration for privacy and interoperability considerations. While technology advances health informatics, our obligation is to ensure prudent and conscientious application, championing ethical care standards and preserving patient wellness.

Biometric Authentication in Health Care Informatics

Unlocking Digital Gates With Identity Verification

Journeying into the fascinating realm of biometrics, unique human characteristics become the key to unlocking the doors of health care data—a personalized handshake with technology whereby human identity converges with the digital landscape. In the symphony of health care informatics, biometrics turns our biological features into the digital keys opening gates to patient records and sensitive health information.

Delving into the layered fortress of authentication beyond the traditional username and password, we add layers involving what you possess—like a smart card or token. The third level—biometrics—introduces technology that recognizes not just what you know and have, but who you are, ensuring a threefold identity check for secure interactions with the healthcare system.

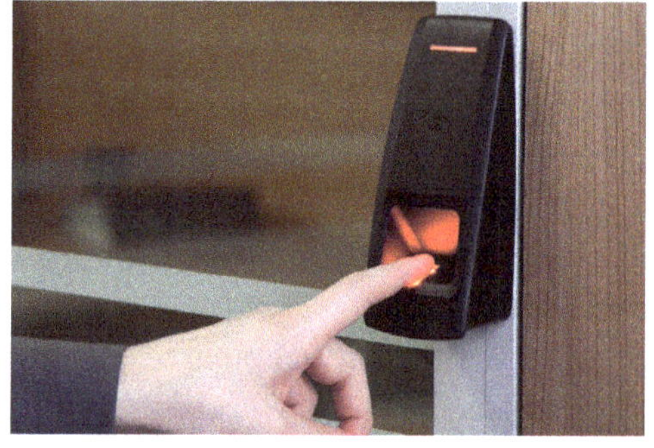

FIGURE 8.2 Biometrics for authentication.

By implementing verification at multiple stages, this method aims to not only safeguard security, but also to guarantee that the individual engaging with the health care system is exactly who they represent themselves as. Each piece of this intricate puzzle—what you know, what you have, and who you are—fits together to grant access, emphasizing a commitment to the ethical stewardship of health care data and preserving patient trust in the digital age.

Summary

As digital health care systems continue to evolve, robust authentication measures remain essential in safeguarding sensitive patient data. By integrating multilayered verification—what you know, what you have, and who you are—this approach strengthens security while ensuring seamless and trustworthy interactions within the health care system. The adoption of biometric authentication alongside traditional methods reflects a commitment to both innovation and ethical data stewardship. Ultimately, these advancements not only protect patient information but also reinforce confidence in the integrity of digital health care, paving the way for a more secure and patient-centric future.

Chapter Review Questions

Directions: Consider what you learned in this chapter as you respond to the health care scenario and questions.

Health Care Scenario: Enhancing Digital Security in Health Care

Dr. Jessica Martinez is a health informatics specialist working at a major urban hospital. Recently, the hospital transitioned from paper-based records to a comprehensive EHR system. Dr. Martinez is tasked with ensuring the security of the hospital's digital health records, identifying potential vulnerabilities, and developing strategies to mitigate cyber threats. She is also responsible for training staff on the importance of digital security and the ethical considerations of handling patient data.

During a recent security audit, Dr. Martinez identified several areas of concern, including weak passwords, lack of multifactor authentication, and outdated encryption protocols. She decides to implement a series of measures to enhance the hospital's digital security, such as upgrading to advanced encryption methods, introducing biometric authentication, and conducting regular training sessions for the staff.

Additionally, Dr. Martinez reviews recent cases of data breaches in other health care institutions to understand the common vulnerabilities and preventive measures. She emphasizes the importance of maintaining data integrity and reliability while ensuring compliance with privacy regulations like HIPAA. Dr. Martinez also explores how the integration of IoT devices and AI-driven analytics can further secure the hospital's digital health environment.

Multiple-Choice Questions

1. What initial step should Dr. Martinez take to identify the hospital's digital security vulnerabilities?
    a. Upgrade encryption methods.
    b. Conduct a security audit.
    c. Implement multifactor authentication.
    d. Train staff on digital security.
2. Which of the following measures is *not* mentioned as a part of Dr. Martinez's security enhancements?
    a. Upgrading encryption methods
    b. Conducting regular staff training sessions
    c. Implementing biometric authentication
    d. Installing new EHR software
3. Why is it important for Dr. Martinez to review recent cases of data breaches in other health care institutions?
    a. To copy their security measures
    b. To understand common vulnerabilities and preventive measures
    c. To identify which hospitals are at risk
    d. To find cheaper security solutions
4. Which technology integration is Dr. Martinez exploring to further secure the hospital's digital health environment?
    a. Virtual reality
    b. IoT devices
    c. Blockchain
    d. Advanced surgical robots

5. How does implementing multifactor authentication enhance the hospital's digital security?
   a. By speeding up the login process
   b. By requiring multiple forms of verification, reducing unauthorized access
   c. By encrypting patient records
   d. By eliminating the need for passwords

6. What is the primary purpose of conducting regular training sessions for the hospital staff?
   a. To teach them how to use new medical equipment
   b. To educate them on the importance of digital security and proper handling of patient data
   c. To train them on advanced surgical techniques
   d. To prepare them for a shift in hospital management

Answer Key

1. (b) Conduct a security audit
2. (d) Installing new EHR software
3. (b) To understand common vulnerabilities and preventive measures
4. (b) IoT devices
5. (b) By requiring multiple forms of verification, reducing unauthorized access
6. (b) To educate them on the importance of digital security and proper handling of patient data

Recommended Reading

IBM. (n.d.). *What is a blockchain?* https://www.ibm.com/blockchain/what-is-blockchain

Orr, D. A., & Lancaster, M. D. (2018). Cryptocurrency and the blockchain: A discussion of forensic need. *International Journal of Cyber-Security and Digital Forensics*, *7*(4), 420–435.

References

Haney, J., & Lutters, W. (2020). Security awareness training for the workforce: Moving beyond "check-the-box" compliance. *Computer, 53*(10). https://doi.org/10.1109/mc.2020.3001959

International Cybersecurity Standardization Working Group. (2015). *Supplemental information for the interagency report on strategic U.S. government engagement in international standardization to achieve U.S. objectives for cybersecurity* (Vol. 2). National Institute of Standards and Technology. http://dx.doi.org/10.6028/NIST.IR.8074v2

Okpara-Oguadimma, A. (2024, March 19). Safeguarding patients' privacy in telehealth: 10 essential privacy and security tips. *HealthCreeks*. https://healthcreeks.com/safeguarding-patients-privacy-in-telehealth-10-essential-privacy-and-security-tips/

Figure Credit

Fig. 8.2: Copyright © by DarienLizard (CC BY-SA 4.0) at https://commons.wikimedia.org/wiki/File:PERCo_CL15_biometric_controller.jpg.

Chapter 9

Designing an Informatics Website

Exploring Principles and Theories of the Field

Introduction

In this chapter, we will embark on an exciting journey that bridges the gap between theory and practice in the realm of nursing informatics. The purpose of Chapter 9 is to show you how the principles and concepts you've learned can be applied in a real-world setting through the development of a comprehensive website. This website will serve as a model, integrating core concepts, principles, and theories of informatics into a valuable resource for graduate-level students, educators, and health professionals.

The significance of Chapter 9 lies in its ability to connect theoretical knowledge with practical application. By engaging in the design of a website, you'll see firsthand how the theories you've studied can be transformed into a functional, digital tool that aids in health care delivery. We will also delve into a case study from a West African village, illustrating the transformative impact of mobile technology on health care. This real-world example not only makes the content relatable but also underscores the importance of informatics in improving health care outcomes in diverse settings.

Through this chapter, you will gain a deeper understanding of the interdisciplinary nature of nursing informatics. You will see how nursing science, computer science, and information science come together to create effective informatics solutions. The website design project exemplifies this integration and demonstrates how these disciplines collaborate to enhance patient care.

As we explore the development of a telehealth or mobile health program, particularly in the context of the West African village, you will be encouraged to think critically about the challenges and opportunities presented by mobile technology. This process will help you develop problem-solving skills as you consider factors such as device selection, workflow optimization, cost reduction, and patient empowerment.

Chapter 9 aims to equip you with the knowledge and skills needed to become effective informatics specialists. By working on this practical project, you will learn how to transform raw data into information, information into knowledge, and knowledge into wisdom. This progression is crucial for improving communication, streamlining data management, and ultimately enhancing patient care.

Objectives That Lead to Outcomes

By clearly distinguishing between process-oriented objectives and result-oriented outcomes, it becomes easier to understand and measure both the actions taken and the results achieved. Thus, the following table aligns key objectives with their corresponding outcomes, providing a clear and detailed understanding of what learners should achieve and comprehend upon completion.

Objective	Outcome
Demonstrate the modeling of key principles in informatics through website design.	The website design effectively incorporates and displays key informatics principles.
Highlight the culmination of core concepts, principles, and theories related to informatics.	The website clearly presents and integrates core informatics concepts, principles, and theories.
Illustrate the understanding of theory, critical thought, and the application of processes in informatics.	The website content demonstrates a deep understanding of informatics theory and practical application.

Provide tangible examples by including pages of the developed website in the chapter.	Specific pages from the website are included as examples in the chapter, showing real-world applications.
Establish the website as a valuable resource for students, educators, and health professionals in the field of informatics.	The website is recognized and utilized as a comprehensive resource by students, educators, and health professionals.
Ensure the website's content is accessible and user-friendly for a diverse audience.	The website's design and content are optimized for accessibility and ease of use, catering to a diverse audience.

Key Terms

Directions: Before reading, please look at this list of key terms that will be used in this chapter. If any term is unfamiliar, please see the glossary at the end of the book.

application of processes
core concepts
critical thought
informatics
key principles
modeling
resource
tangible examples pages of the website
theories
website design

Constructing a Patient-Centered Program

Guided by Nursing and Health Care Informatics Principles and Technology Integration

Armed with a commitment to health care, a vision for technology integration, and an unwavering focus on patient centered care, we embark on the development of the program using mobile phone units for remote monitoring, cloud technology, and a commitment to keeping it patient centered. For nurse informatics graduate students, we apply functioning tenets sourced from the American Nurses Association's standards of practice for informatics nurses.

These serve as a compass for the varied journeys we undertake to make meaningful use of technology. As we explore options for remote monitoring, we realize the importance of choosing what is accessible to the community, acknowledging the potential impact of our choices.

Harnessing Technology for Longevity: The HGFLP Approach

The Health Guardian for Longevity Program (HGFLP) leverages technology, mobile solutions, cloud computing, and communication platforms to achieve its objectives. These integrated components enhance accessibility, streamline data management, and facilitate seamless communication, all aimed at improving health outcomes and promoting longevity.

Figure 9.1 illustrates the key goals of the HGFLP and how its core components—technology, mobile solutions, cloud computing, and communication platforms—contribute to achieving them.

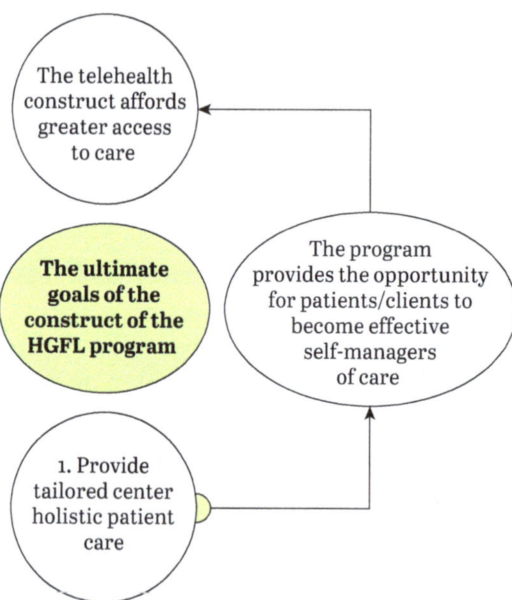

FIGURE 9.1 Goals of the HGFL program.

Components of the Program

Technology, Mobile, Cloud, and Communication Platform

Let us dive into the program's components: technology, mobile, cloud, and the communication platform. These deliberate choices serve as the building blocks of our program, and as we continue to work on it, we anticipate exciting developments. Stay tuned as the journey unfolds, weaving together theory, critical thought, and real-world application in the dynamic landscape of nursing and health care informatics.

Foundational Theories

Building the Conceptual Framework for the HGFLP

Along this journey, engaging questions will periodically emerge for your contemplation. Our first task is to lay the groundwork by sharing the theories that form the conceptual framework for the HGFLP. Shaping the program has been an evolving process, influenced by key studies and insights from research. In 2012, West's (2012) research illuminated the potential of remote monitoring technology, suggesting substantial savings over 25 years. Telenor Group's findings in 2011 displayed the benefits of mobile technology, particularly for the older population. These insights played a pivotal role in the mission to empower the elderly and expectant mothers in underserved areas.

Contributing to the program's construction, a key study by Quest in 2010 highlighted the role of mobile technology in chronic disease management. This resulted in a vision to improve health outcomes and medical efficiency, utilizing remote monitoring for patients in underserved communities.

Statistics further fueled the commitment as alarming trends were observed, particularly in West Africa, where an average lifespan of 50 to 60 years was deemed unacceptable. Motivated by these challenges, a 501(c)(3) charity was established in 2010 to address persistent issues and ensure regular assessments.

Community Overview

Size, Health Care Model, Health Care Challenges, and Financial Constraints

The case study on the HGFLP delves into a community of approximately 30,000 residents facing health care challenges due to financial constraints (Pemberton, 2021). Despite government efforts, accessibility remains a significant hurdle, and the case study explores the impact of advancements, geographic context, and ongoing development on health care accessibility. We zoom in on the specific challenges faced by the community, particularly dietary constraints dominated by high-carb cornmeal.

Concerns about hypoglycemia, hyperglycemia, and potential implications for type II diabetes in children highlight the need for intervention. Acknowledging the complexity, we explore practical solutions, emphasizing the importance of addressing nutritional aspects. Poor nutrition emerges as a significant contributor to the

Summary of Assessed Data

School Age (6-10)
N = 9
Females = 6
Males = 3

Ref. Normal B/P 97-115/57-76
Hypotension = 5 Females B/Ps 80/40, 87/37, 86/48,82/42, 96/44
Hypotension = 2 Males 95/56, 88/49

Pulse: **Elevated Pulse**
2 Females 110
Oxygen Sat. Low 73 (M) and 64 (F)
Hyperglycemia = 3 Females Levels 199, 148, 131, 127
Hyperglycemia = 1 Male 133
Hypoglycemia - = 1 Male 41
Hypoglycemia = 1 Female 46

Adolescent Age (13-18)
N = 6
ALL Females

Ref. Normal B/P is 110-131/64-83

Hypotension = 1
B/P 92/50
Hypertension = 1
B/P 147/95
Hypoglycemic = 1
Hyperglycemic = 1

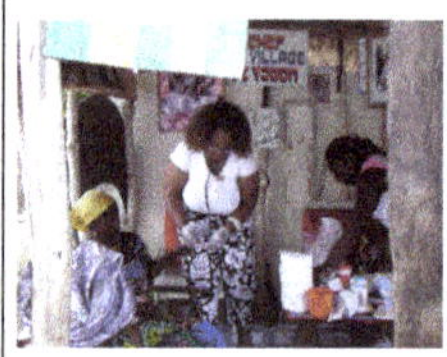

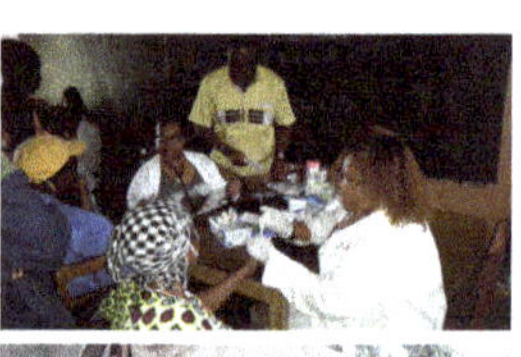

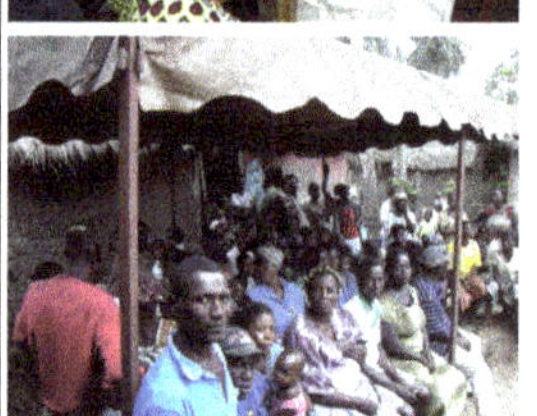

FIGURE 9.2 Rising demand for telehealth.

community's shortened lifespan, compounded by late diagnoses and delayed interventions. Our commitment is unwavering as we transition from qualitative to quantitative analysis, aiming to make a substantial impact on eradicating these issues.

The narrative unfolds with a holistic health assessment and collaborative effort involving health care providers and commissioners from the village. We take a comprehensive approach, covering physical, mental, environmental, and spiritual aspects. Challenges arise, prompting a shift in our approach toward sustainability in health care delivery, ensuring enduring health outcomes for the community.

Summary of Assessed Data

Young Adult Age (19-40)	**Middle Adult Age (42-65)**	**Older Adult Age (65+)**
N = 38	N = 37	N = 10,
Females = 26	Females = 24	Females = 6 Males =4
Males = 12	Male = 13	
HTN = 4 Males	**HTN** = 11 Females	**HTN** = 5 Females
HTN = 2 Females	**HTN** = 7 Males	**HTN** = 1 Male
	Hypotension = 1 Female	
B/P 184/135 (M), 156/82(M), 147/83(M), 203/132 (F), 176/112(M), 158/99 (F)	**B/Ps:** 175/126(M), 149/95(F), 162/87(M), 154/90(F), 157/84 (M), 163/90 (F), 153/78(F), 172/93 (F), 185/108(F), 165/107(M), 150/72(F), 154/76(M),168/93 (F), 162/87(F), 166/83(M), 142/101(F), 151/70(F)	**B/Ps:** F192/92, 189/127, 174/93, 153/93, 150/80 M163/101
Pulse: elevated 2 Females 110	**Pulse: High** Male 129, Female 114	**Pulse:** Low Male 50
O_2 Saturation: Low 73(M) and 64 (F)	**O_2 Saturation:** 95(M), 94(M), 95(F), 93(F), 94(M), 96(F)	**O_2 Saturation:** normal (ALL)
Glucose: Low 41 (M), 46 (F) **High** 127 (F), 131 (F), 133 (M), 148 (F), 199 (F)	**Glucose:** Low 48(M), 59(M), High 213(F), 178(F), 199 (F)	**Glucose:** High 134 (M), 124 (F)
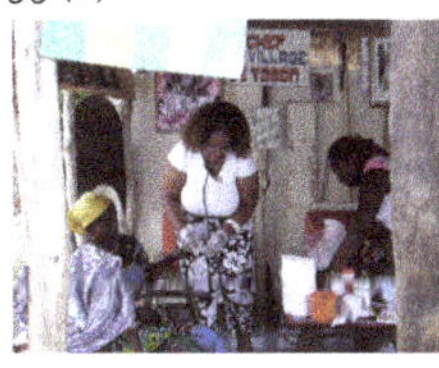	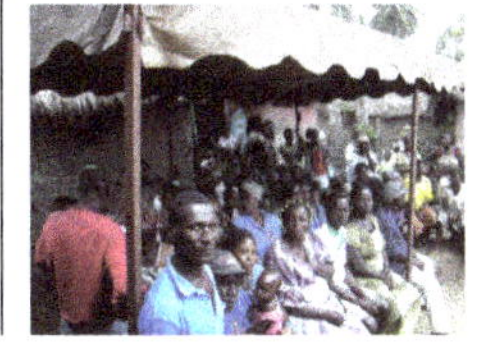	

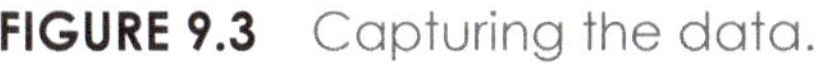

FIGURE 9.3 Capturing the data.

As we delve deeper into the transformative power of technology and health care interventions, stay tuned for the unfolding narrative of the HGFLP, a testament to the resilience of communities, the power of informed choices, and the impact of holistic health care initiatives.

For school-age children and adolescents, hypertension, hypotension, and hyperglycemia emerged as significant concerns, necessitating a more sustained and impactful intervention strategy. For adults of varying age ranges, from 19 to 44, middle-aged adults (42 to 65), and older adults (65 and above), the spotlight intensifies to understand and address their unique health challenges (Pemberton, 2021).

Our commitment extends beyond immediate health stabilization. Identifying deficiencies prompts a reconsideration of our approach, ensuring interventions lead to lasting improvements for the residents of the village.

Reflecting on the highlighted health issues, particularly elevated blood pressures across age groups, emphasizes the urgency of our intervention. Hypertension spans from young adults to the elderly, underscoring the necessity for a timely and impactful program. A poignant incident of a young man suffering a stroke highlights the potential benefits of earlier intervention.

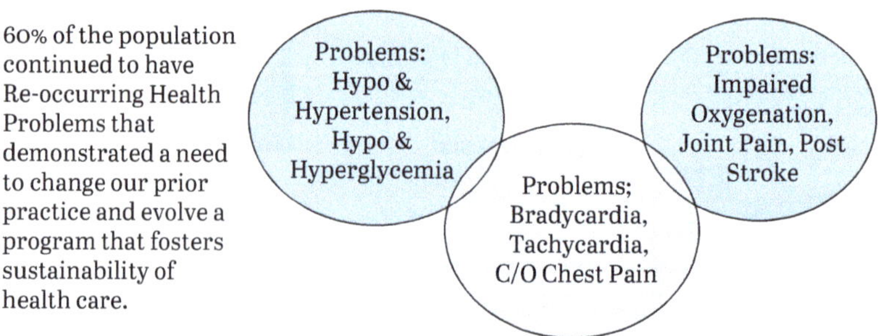

FIGURE 9.4 Significance of the problem.

Empowering Communities

Objectives of the HGFLP

Transitioning into the objectives of the HGFLP, our aim is clear: Address and rectify health challenges through restoration and sustained healthy practices. The program's objective is to empower participants by deepening their understanding of disease, treatment, recovery, and maintenance processes (Pemberton, 2017). Team leaders act as liaisons, fostering direct communication with the population, making participants effective managers of their care within the convenience of their village.

Incorporating modified mobile technology to account for virtual access constraints, the program enhances coping skills, reduces stress, and facilitates holistic health behaviors. Humor videos, integrated into the community website, add a touch of lightness to the program, emphasizing the importance of a holistic approach to health.

The foundation of the program lies in a better understanding of diagnosis, treatment, and recovery, coupled with robust support systems. Root causes of health issues are assessed, strategies are developed, and information and computer sciences components are incorporated for a comprehensive approach (Pemberton, 2021). By adapting the U.S. model to West Africa, we acknowledge the challenges but remain steadfast in our commitment to bringing sustainable health improvements to the same village.

Navigating

Exploration of Website Pages

In exploring the interactive features of the HGFLP, we delve into a demo website designed for sustainable health improvements. The website serves as a valuable resource, introducing users to the program's background, objectives, key issues, and interactive features.

Demonstrating a setup similar to our practices in the United States, the program extends a supportive approach to the community in West Africa. Navigation buttons guide users through sections covering heart health, theoretical explanations, and intervention plans, ensuring continuous support through a dedicated section for conference calls. Humor videos add a touch of lightness to the

THE MAJOR OBJECTIVES OF THE HGFLP

- Facilitate restoration and sustain health behavioral practices using a tailored health care approach that incorporates mobile technology.
- Enhance patients'/consumers' understanding of the disease, treatment, recovery, and maintenance.
- Empower patients/consumers to be key players in self-care after diagnosis or crisis.
- Empower patients/consumers to become effective managers of their care in a favorable environment or convenience and comfort.
- Enhance coping skills.
- Facilitate holistic healthy behaviors with a touch of humor both nationally and internationally.

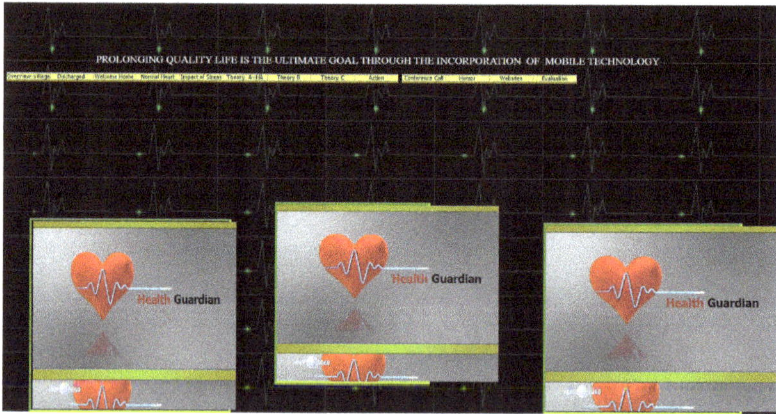

FIGURE 9.5 Demo: HGFLP.

educational content, making the program engaging. Regular updates reflect progress, and, leveraging technology, content is distributed to the village via flash drives for continuous learning.

The program's success is evaluated through client feedback and case study analyses, ensuring its adaptability to evolving community needs. This comprehensive approach aligns with the goal of enhancing participants' understanding and empowering them to manage their health effectively. The website serves as a dynamic platform, evolving with the progress of the community and embodying the principles discussed in the narrative.

As we delve deeper into the program, our commitment to participant engagement becomes apparent. The program goes beyond theoretical education and intervention and incorporates interactive activities that cater to different audiences, including children. Leveraging the internet, we integrate gaming instructional activities and content from reputable sources like Medline Plus. This streamlined approach provides participants with a wealth of information without the need for redundant applications.

The website's modular structure allows users to explore topics at their own pace, ensuring personalized learning experiences. Stress reduction is a key focus, highlighted through a 24/7 support system featuring a videoconference call feature. The program emphasizes meeting the community where they are most comfortable, utilizing various platforms for accessibility. Instructional pieces on the website, accompanied by music and relatable content, contribute to a comfortable and motivating learning environment.

Humor plays a pivotal role in making the content engaging, as seen in the humorous video and instructional pieces on stress reduction. This creative instructive approach, often contributed by my students specializing in informatics, enhances the relatability of the content and diversifies ideas. The program integrates theoretical knowledge, interactive activities, and continuous support to empower participants in managing their health effectively. The modular website design, coupled with multimedia elements, creates a dynamic and engaging learning environment aligned with the program's objectives and principles. This collaborative effort contributes to the diversity of ideas and efficiency in content creation.

Implementation Methodology and Team Involvement

The implementation involved assessing 200 individuals, with 100 randomly selected for the study. To ease the workload on team leaders, participants were divided into age-based groups. Team leaders, acting as liaisons, played a crucial role in maintaining communication with participants (Pemberton, 2021).

Instructions were provided to both the community and team leaders, emphasizing a clear understanding and consistent implementation of the program. The qualitative design adopted in the initial phase focused on gathering feedback to shape the program's adaptation and refinement.

Results Guided by Logic Model

Guided by a logic model, the results of the qualitative design influenced the study's direction, ensuring alignment with the community's needs. This iterative process facilitates continuous improvement and adaptation based on received feedback.

Study Evaluation and Key Questions

Key questions were addressed in the study evaluation, focusing on the HGFL program's effectiveness in meeting objectives. The assessment included the impact of humor videos, effectiveness of videoconference calls, and comparison to prior on-site programs. Participants' feedback indicated positive responses, with the program design, background, and music being well received.

Despite positive feedback, recommendations for further modification were considered, particularly in team leader and participant training to bridge language barriers. Acknowledging language differences as a challenge, ongoing efforts were recognized to address this aspect of the program.

Looking ahead, the program addresses concerns about remote monitoring with the introduction of varied devices. Celler et al. (2003) designed a remote device for patients to manage chronic diseases at home, which incorporates various instruments empowering individuals to monitor and manage their health effectively. The transition to remote monitoring reflects the program's commitment to staying at the forefront of health care innovations for lasting impact.

Demonstration of Branko's Device Capabilities

A demonstration of Professor Branko's remote monitoring device reveals the program's capabilities in spirometry for lung function analysis and ECG recording. The device features a comprehensive audio-visual communication system, medication management, questionnaires, and a health diary aiming to facilitate efficient data exchange and appointment scheduling and to address health concerns.

Revolutionizing Patient Care

Exploring the Transformative Power of Information and Communications Technology

The potential impact on patient care and management becomes evident as the presenter explores the functionalities of information and communications technology (ICT). Real-time monitoring and seamless interaction with health care professionals are emphasized, simplifying the user experience for those who may not be comfortable with typing.

Negotiations surrounding the costs of the device are acknowledged, recognizing the financial considerations despite the association with a public charity. The presenter's story about seeking permission for a costly anatomical heart illustration reflects the ongoing efforts to enhance the program's capabilities and bridge gaps in health care accessibility.

Practical aspects of implementing remote monitoring devices, such as ICT, are considered, highlighting challenges like device cost and the necessity of Wi-Fi connections. Fortunately, the village in Benin collaborating with the teams already has Wi-Fi infrastructure, highlighting technological progress since the presenter's initial visit in 2001.

Logistics of Distributing the Program

Logistics of distributing the program are discussed, with flash drives sent to team leaders who play a pivotal role in disseminating information within the village. Language barriers remain a challenge, and the presenter emphasizes the importance of team leaders as communicators for the presenter and the community.

The role of team leaders in addressing language barriers and facilitating effective communication is highlighted. Peer support within the same language and cultural background is considered, with team leaders acting as navigators and recording patient concerns for communication with the presenter.

The importance of refining the interpretive piece is emphasized, recognizing the ongoing challenge of language barriers. The discussion takes an interesting turn as concerns about language barriers transforming information accurately are addressed, emphasizing the need for specialized interpreters in medical contexts

Role of Team Leaders and Language Barriers

Clarifications about the professionalism of team leaders dispel misconceptions about their medical expertise. Questions about understanding health problems in the village, particularly related to food habits, lead to discussions about cultural shifts, positive changes in vegetable production, and concerns about costs.

The role of the government and potential obstacles in implementing health initiatives are explored. The presenter's personal journey from trauma critical care to utilizing technology for health initiatives adds a human touch to the narrative, providing context to their expertise and dedication.

In summary, the discussion covers language translation challenges, the professional background of team leaders, cultural shifts in food habits, concerns about costs, the role of the government, and the presenter's personal journey. The challenges and complexities faced underscore the dedication required in implementing effective health care solutions in diverse contexts.

Summary

This chapter has traversed through the foundational building blocks, insightful research contributions, and the intricate details of a case study in West Africa. Core concepts, principles, and theories related to informatics were demonstrated through the development of a website. The program, shaped by deliberate choices in technology, mobile, cloud, and communication platforms, stands as a beacon of transformative health care initiatives.

Our narrative unfolded with the exploration of theoretical frameworks, impactful studies, and statistical realities, driving the establishment of a program dedicated to extending lifespans in underserved communities. The case study delved into the challenges of health care accessibility, government efforts, and the promising impact of technological advancements.

The chapter homed in on specific challenges faced by the community, particularly dietary constraints that have implications. The commitment to addressing poor nutrition, late diagnoses, and limited access to health promotion programs fueled the mission of the HGFLP.

Overall, Chapter 9 delved into the holistic health assessment, collaborative efforts, and the practical implementation of the program. We witnessed the program's evolution from qualitative to quantitative analysis, emphasizing the transformative power of technology and health care interventions.

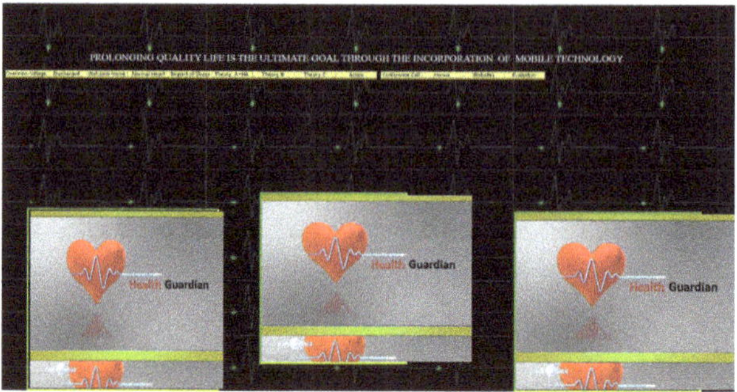

Home page

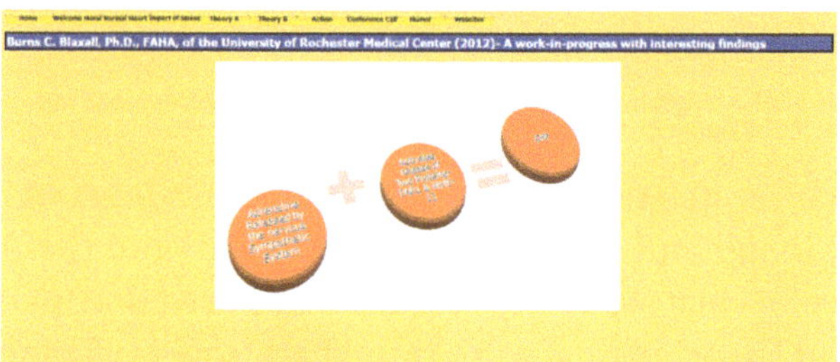

Sample Theory of Health Issue

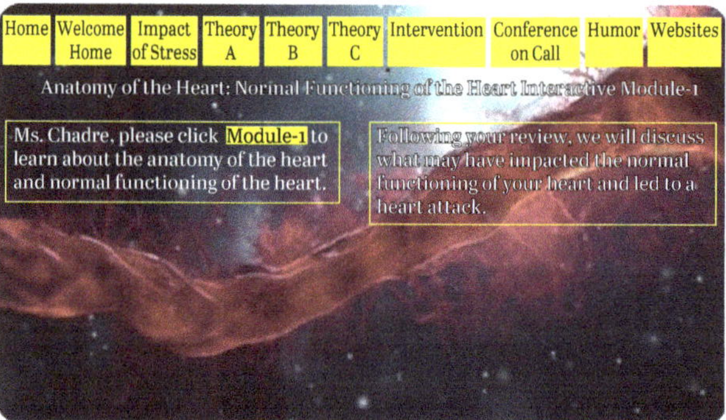

Sample Interactive page

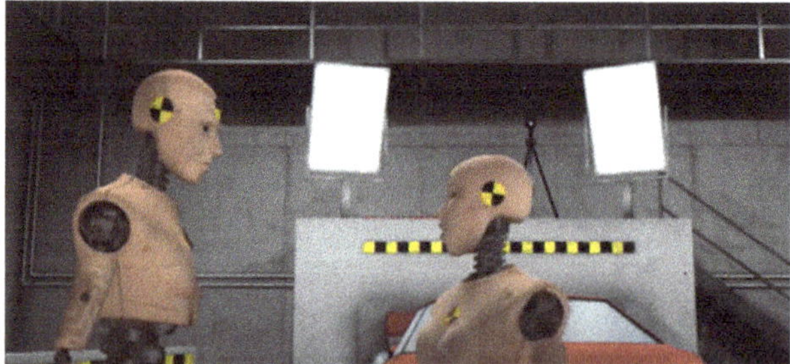

Sample Humor Video by Student

FIGURE 9.6 Sample Website Pages for Illustration

Chapter Review Questions

Directions: Consider what you learned in this chapter as you respond to the health care scenario and questions.

Health Care Scenario: Designing an Informatics Website and Exploring Principles and Theories of the Field

You are part of a team tasked with developing a telehealth platform for a remote village in West Africa. The village lacks consistent access to health care facilities, and mobile technology offers a promising solution to bridge this gap. Your team's goal is to design a website that integrates telehealth services tailored to the community's needs, promoting better health outcomes through improved access to medical advice and remote monitoring.

Multiple-Choice Questions

1. What is the primary objective of developing the telehealth platform for the West African village?

    a. Improve access to health care facilities.
    b. Provide digital entertainment options.
    c. Enhance communication with friends.
    d. Expand agricultural knowledge.

2. Which interdisciplinary skills are most critical for the successful implementation of the telehealth platform?

    a. Engineering and geology
    b. Nursing science and computer science
    c. Political science and philosophy
    d. Literature and art history

3. Why is mobile technology particularly suited for addressing health care challenges in remote areas like the West African village?

    a. It requires minimal infrastructure investment.
    b. It can only be used in urban environments.

   c. It relies on fixed broadband connections.
   d. It is costly and difficult to maintain.

4. What are some key considerations when selecting mobile devices for the telehealth platform?

   a. High cost and complex design
   b. Compatibility with local languages and ease of use
   c. Limited battery life and low screen resolution
   d. Limited functionality and high data usage

5. How does the telehealth platform contribute to patient empowerment in the West African village?

   a. By restricting access to medical information
   b. By requiring constant in-person consultations
   c. By enabling self-care management and access to medical advice
   d. By limiting communication between patients and health care providers

6. What potential challenges might arise during the implementation of the telehealth platform in the West African village?

   a. Language barriers and cultural differences
   b. Overabundance of health care facilities
   c. Excessive government regulation
   d. Limited access to mobile devices

Answer Key

1. (a) Improve access to health care facilities.
2. (b) Nursing science and computer science
3. (a) It requires minimal infrastructure investment.
4. (b) Compatibility with local languages and ease of use
5. (c) By enabling self-care management and access to medical advice
6. (a) Language barriers and cultural differences

Recommended Reading

Gustafson, D.H., Hawkins, R., Boberg, E., Pingree, S., Serlin, R.E., Graziano, F., & Chan, C.L. (1999). Impact of a patient- centered, computer-based health information/support system. *American Journal of Preventative Medicine, 16*(1):1–9. doi: 10.1016/s0749-3797(98)00108-1. PMID: 9894548.

Jenny, N. Y. Y., & Fai, T. S. (2001). Evaluating the effectiveness of an interactive multimedia computer-based patient education program in cardiac rehabilitation. *Occupational Therapy Journal of Research*, *21*(4), 260–275.

Telenor Group. (2018). *Realizing digital Myanmar: Leapfrogging to an inclusive digital economy*. https://www.telenor.com/wp-content/uploads/2018/02/Telenor-Realising-Digital-Myanmar-Report-06-February.

World Health Organization. (n.d.). *Benin*. https://www.who.int/data/gho/data/countries/country-details/GHO/benin

References

American Nurses Association. (2022). *Nursing informatics scope and standards of practice*.

Celler, B.G., Lovell, N. H., & Basilakis, J. (2003). Using information technology to improve the management of chronic disease. *Medical Journal of Australia*, *179*(5), 242–246.

Pemberton, F. (2017). A tailored approach is key: The Health Guardian for Longevity Program uses mobile technology to sustain healthy life behaviors. *COJ Nursing & Healthcare*, *1*(1), Article COJNH.000501. https://doi.org/10.31031/COJNH.2017.01.000501

Pemberton, F. (2021). Village participants' perceptions on the use of the Health Guardian for Longevity Program to sustain health in West Africa. *COJ Nursing & Healthcare*, *7*(3). https://doi.org/10.31031/COJNH.2021.07.000665

West, D. M. (2012). How mobile devices are transforming healthcare. *Issues in Technology Innovation*, (18), 1–14. https://www.brookings.edu/research/how-mobile-devices-are-transforming-healthcare/

Figure Credits

Chapter 10

Keeping Up With the Advancements in Technology

Introduction

The purpose of Chapter 10 is to take everything learned so far and apply it to real-world scenarios. One of our key objectives is to implement telemedicine solutions to expand access to health care services, which will enable remote consultations and monitoring, ultimately improving patient care. Another important goal is to integrate e-learning platforms to enhance the delivery of educational content, making learning more accessible and engaging for students. We will also focus on developing and deploying a user-friendly telehealth platform, ensuring seamless remote health care interactions while prioritizing patient privacy and security.

Moreover, we aim to enhance homecare services through the integration of smart home technologies, providing support for daily activities and health monitoring for individuals receiving care at home. Additionally, fostering innovation and creativity by establishing a platform for independent technology projects will encourage and support employees and students in contributing to the organization's overall technological advancement. Finally, we will create a centralized repository of models representing completed technological projects, serving as a valuable resource for knowledge sharing and reference within the organization or institution.

The significance of Chapter 10 lies in its focus on practical application. After laying a strong theoretical foundation in the previous chapters, in this chapter theory meets practice. By implementing telemedicine, developing e-learning platforms, and enhancing homecare through smart technologies, students will see firsthand how informatics can transform health care delivery and education. This chapter also emphasizes the importance of innovation and creativity, encouraging students to apply their knowledge in ways that drive technological advancement. Additionally, creating a centralized repository for technological projects ensures that knowledge and innovations are shared and accessible, fostering a collaborative learning environment.

Foundations from Chapters 1 through 9

In Chapter 1, we set the stage by defining the scope and significance of informatics in the health care domain. Subsequent chapters delved into fundamental concepts, from data management strategies (Chapter 2) to the intricacies of HCIS (Chapter 3). Chapters 4 and 5 took us into the realms of interoperability and standards, emphasizing the importance of seamless data exchange in modern health care ecosystems. Building on this, Chapter 6 explored the ethical considerations inherent in managing health information. Chapter 7 brought us face-to-face with the challenges and opportunities of data analytics in health care, offering a glimpse into the power of insights derived from vast datasets. Chapter 8 delved into the critical realm of cybersecurity, recognizing the paramount importance of safeguarding patient information in our interconnected world. The culmination of our theoretical journey occurred in Chapter 9, where website design became a dynamic canvas for implementing key informatics principles. This digital creation not only displayed theoretical understanding but also served as a tangible representation of the advanced skill set acquired by graduate-level informatics students.

Transition to Chapter 10

We have reached a pivotal phase. Chapter 9 focused on the practical implementation of key principles through the intricate process of website design. This endeavor was not just an exercise in technical application but also a sophisticated demonstration of theoretical understanding, critical thinking, and the adept utilization of informatics methodologies.

This statement of purpose and significance for Chapter 10 is designed to not only solidify your theoretical knowledge but also to empower you with practical skills that can drive significant advancements in health care and education through innovative informatics solutions.

Objectives That Lead to Outcomes

Specific objectives and their corresponding expected outcomes are outlined for this chapter. The following table aligns key objectives with their outcomes, providing a clear and detailed understanding of what learners should achieve and comprehend upon completion. This alignment ensures that each objective is met with a tangible and measurable outcome, enhancing the overall learning experience. These objectives will guide the planning and execution of the HIS project, ensuring it aligns with the organization's strategic goals and principles of effective project management and organizational management.

Objective	Outcome
Implement telemedicine solutions to expand access to health care services.	Remote consultations and monitoring improve patient care.
Integrate e-learning platforms to enhance the delivery of educational content.	Learning becomes more accessible and engaging for students.
Develop and deploy a user-friendly telehealth platform.	Ensure seamless remote health care interactions, prioritizing patient privacy and security.
Enhance homecare services through the integration of smart home technologies.	Provide support for daily activities and health monitoring for individuals receiving care at home.
Foster innovation and creativity by establishing a platform for independent technology projects.	Encourage and support employees/students in contributing to the organization's overall technological advancement.
Create a centralized repository of models representing completed technological projects.	Serve as a valuable resource for knowledge sharing and reference within the organization or institution.

Key Terms

Directions: Before reading, please look at this list of key terms that will be used in this chapter. If any term is unfamiliar, please see the glossary at the end of the book.

artificial intelligence
e-learning
homecare
machine learning
remote monitoring

Intellectual Journey

The focus in this chapter sharpens the exploration of cutting-edge technological programs actively shaping health care interventions. This chapter is curated to challenge and engage health care informatics students with innovative solutions. The commitment to sustainable health improvements, particularly for marginalized communities, remains at the forefront. In essence, this chapter beckons the health care informatics student to a heightened level of discourse and exploration. It extends an invitation to delve deeper into the evolving landscape of technology in health care, aligning with the advanced perspectives and aspirations inherent in graduate-level studies.

Equitable Health Advancements

The advancements we explore aim not only to push the boundaries of technology but also to make a meaningful impact on the lives of those facing barriers to quality health care. In essence, this chapter unfolds as a synthesis of our cumulative knowledge, serving as a gateway to the evolving landscape of technology in health care. We are poised to become active contributors to the ongoing narrative of health care informatics, embodying the advanced perspectives and aspirations inherent in our academic journey.

In the rapidly evolving landscape of health care informatics, graduate students find themselves at the head of a technological revolution. The integration of AI, ML, and smart data analysis has reshaped how we approach patient care and manage health care on a global scale. This seismic shift is evident in transformative applications such as personalized medicine and advanced diagnostics.

Take, for instance, the realm of personalized medicine, where AI delves into a patient's genetic code, lifestyle habits, and medical history to construct personalized treatment plans. This level of precision not only enhances treatment efficacy but also minimizes adverse effects and optimizes the allocation of health care resources. Similarly, envision AI algorithms scrutinizing medical imaging, such as MRI or CT scans, catching early signs of illnesses like growths that could pose serious threats.

As health care becomes more intertwined with technology, the connection between health and learning grows clearer. AR/VR technologies are bringing medical education to life, creating immersive learning experiences for students. Telehealth, extending care and knowledge across geographical distances, is breaking barriers and emphasizing the importance of this blend between health care and technology.

Looking ahead, the future of health care informatics holds promises of groundbreaking changes. Genomic studies, personalized medicine plans, and the integration of blockchain technology are poised to revolutionize the approach to treatment. To navigate this future landscape successfully, health care informatics scholars must not only hone their technical skills but also develop a keen understanding of the ethical considerations surrounding health care technology.

In this chapter, we continue to delve into the essential skills for success in health care informatics, emphasizing the need for effective communication and collaboration. Further, protecting patient details and ensuring unbiased code are not just professional obligations but moral imperatives ingrained in the very fabric of the health care informatics role.

The next stage in health care involves the seamless integration of emerging technologies like IoT-supported wearable sensor devices, AI, and blockchain. Remarkably, the widespread adoption of smart wearable sensors is driving a transformation in health care, moving it away from a traditional hub-based system to a more personalized health care management system (HMS; Junaid et al., 2022).

Unveiling the Technological Horizon

As technological advancements reshape the health care ecosystem, the ability to adapt to constant shifts becomes a key determinant of success. Ethical considerations take center stage in the era of data dominance, emphasizing the moral imperatives ingrained in the health care informatics role.

Students find themselves at the forefront of a profound technological revolution. AI, ML, and smart data analysis have fundamentally reshaped patient care and global health care management. This transformative shift is evident in applications like personalized medicine and advanced diagnostics. Previous chapters illustrated AI and ML advancements in health care, offering a deeper understanding of their impact on personalized medicine, diagnostics, predictive analytics, and virtual health assistants. This humanized approach underscores tangible benefits for patient outcomes and overall health care accessibility.

Expanding beyond health care, the transition to the educational realm reveals how AI and ML continue to revolutionize learning experiences. Adaptive learning platforms, intelligent tutoring systems, automated grading, and predictive analytics display transformative potential in education, necessitating enhancements in student engagement and personalized learning experiences.

Our journey concludes with a reflection on the interconnectedness of AI and ML advancements in both health care and education. It offers glimpses into the future, emphasizing health care informatics' real-world impact through cutting-edge technologies and products.

Stemming from previous efforts to enhance patient care, particularly in home settings, the introduction of smart home technologies aligns with the health care profession's commitment to providing holistic care. This leverages technology to support daily activities and remotely monitor health for individuals receiving care at home. This chapter's objective formalizes and supports independent technology projects. This recognizes the importance of individual initiatives in contributing to the organization's overall technological advancement.

Assignment 1: Addressing Holistic Health Care Through Knowledge Application

As we approach the culmination website project, students are entrusted with the creation of a professional website designed to tackle a multifaceted social crisis. The primary objective is to deliver preventive health care education via both asynchronized and synchronized platforms. The website is anticipated to effectively respond to health care needs stemming from adverse events, leveraging the knowledge acquired through readings in subsequent chapters. Additionally, enhance your knowledge of product solutions

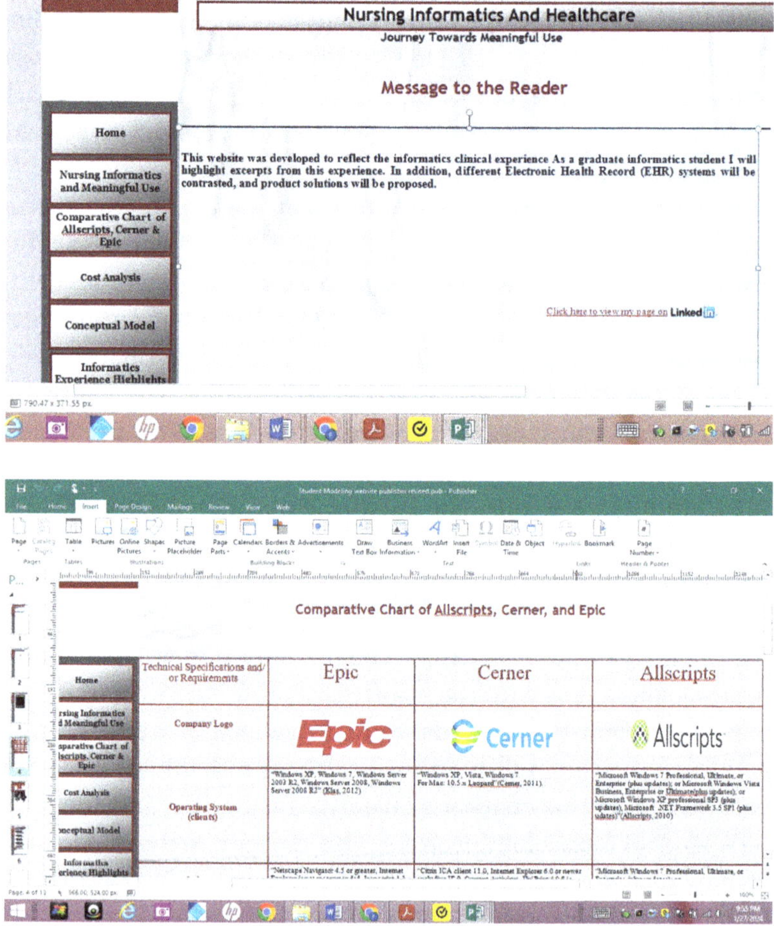

FIGURE 10.1 Sample cost analysis and comparative chart.

used in practice by incorporating a conceptual model for three HIT systems relevant to the project or, alternatively, develop your own product using available construction resources.

To support the project, students will create a comparative chart showcasing the features of the three product solutions, preparing it for presentation to a mock board of directors. This will be followed by a comprehensive cost analysis chart tailored to the proposed solutions, ensuring financial feasibility and alignment with the project's objectives. The website will be enriched with meaningful graphics, images, videos, apps, and interactive resources to maximize engagement and effectiveness.

Beyond education, the website will also serve as a foundation for a health promotion program designed to address the needs of the targeted community affected by the adverse life situation. A database will be incorporated to capture demographics and vital information about the focus group, emphasizing relevant elements necessary for effective intervention.

To assess the website's impact, students will integrate an evaluation survey to gather participants' responses to both the website and the health promotion program. Additionally, as part of the modeling process, students will develop and embed an original, meaningful humor video to engage users and enhance interaction.

As health care informatics students, you will independently determine the issue you wish to address, applying critical thinking and creativity to develop innovative solutions. The following box provides examples for inspiration.

List of Culminating Ideas for Project Development

In today's interconnected world, addressing pressing global challenges requires innovative approaches and comprehensive strategies. This list highlights key areas of focus for project development, ranging from public health crises and environmental impacts to advancements in technology and cultural integration.

- Post COVID-19 pandemic
- Lead found in Flint, Michigan, and Newark, New Jersey, water
- Chronic health problems noted as major health issues nationally and internationally

- Mental and behavioral health issues worldwide
- Bridging cultures worldwide
- Impact of natural disasters
- High rates of maternal mortality and morbidity
- Global event project
- Health disparities
- AI in practice, education, administration

Assignment 2: Community Health Outreach Program

Step 1: Create a digital registration form.

> Application: Utilize a user-friendly digital platform to design a comprehensive registration form.
>
> Alignment: This form will serve as a crucial tool to capture pertinent data, including household income, ensuring a holistic understanding of the community's needs.

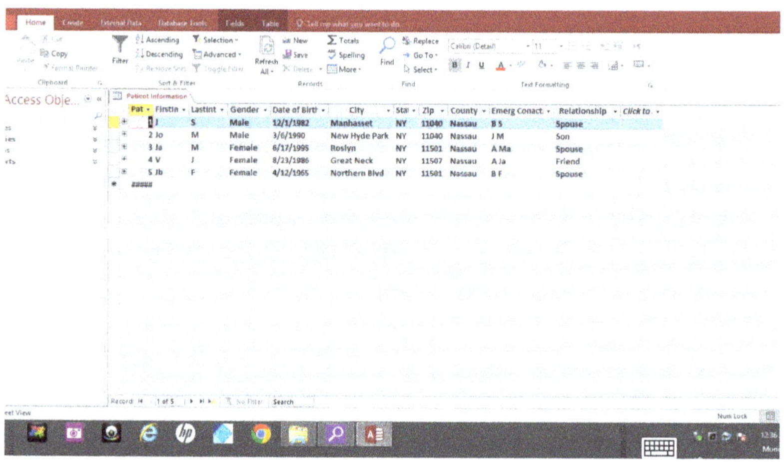

Pat	FirstIn	LastInt	Gender	Date of Birth	City	Stat	Zip	County	Emerg Conact	Relationship	Click to
1	J	S	Male	12/1/1982	Manhasset	NY	11040	Nassau	B S	Spouse	
2	Jo	M	Male	3/6/1990	New Hyde Park	NY	11040	Nassau	J M	Son	
3	Ja	M	Female	6/17/1995	Roslyn	NY	11501	Nassau	A Ma	Spouse	
4	V	J	Female	8/23/1986	Great Neck	NY	11507	Nassau	A Ja	Friend	
5	Jb	F	Female	4/12/1965	Northern Blvd	NY	11501	Nassau	B F	Spouse	

FIGURE 10.2 Capture data using access.

Step 2: Research lead poisoning and educational YouTube creation.

> Application: Conduct thorough research on lead poisoning, emphasizing its impact on children.

Alignment: Develop an engaging YouTube video that educates the community on lead poisoning, with a particular focus on the sequence of long-term care. Ensure the content emphasizes periodic follow-ups for sustained health.

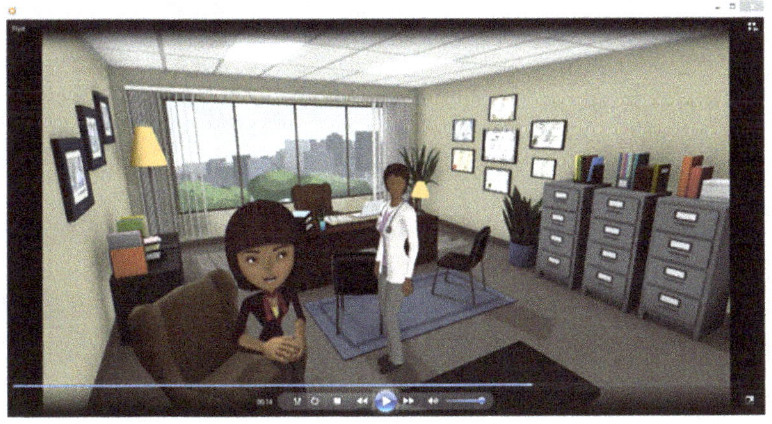

FIGURE 10.3 Addressing the Flint situation.

Step 3: Reach out to a family impacted by the Flint situation.

Application: Establish direct communication with a family affected by the Flint water crisis.

Alignment: Organize a videoconference session to empathetically understand their situation, needs, and concerns.

Step 4: Set goals and create virtual access.

Application: Collaborate with the impacted family to set achievable health-related goals.

Alignment: Develop a dedicated website offering virtual/mobile access to health-related information, resources, and support tailored to the family's needs.

Grocery List

Product	Cost	Nutritional Value
Peanut Butter	$0.99	
Jam/Jelly	$0.99	
Canned Tuna	$0.59	
Chicken	$0.89/lbs	
Frozen Mixed Vegetables	$0.99	
Frozen Mixed Fruits	$0.99	

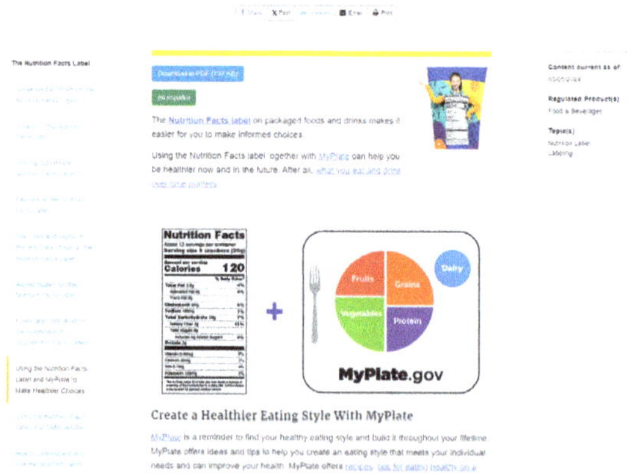

FIGURE 10.4 Nutrition teaching tool creation.

Step 5: Create educational humor videos.

Application: Leverage creative skills to produce humorous educational videos.

Alignment: These videos should serve not only to entertain but also to reinforce the idea that access to care is readily available. Emphasize a positive and approachable atmosphere for seeking assistance.

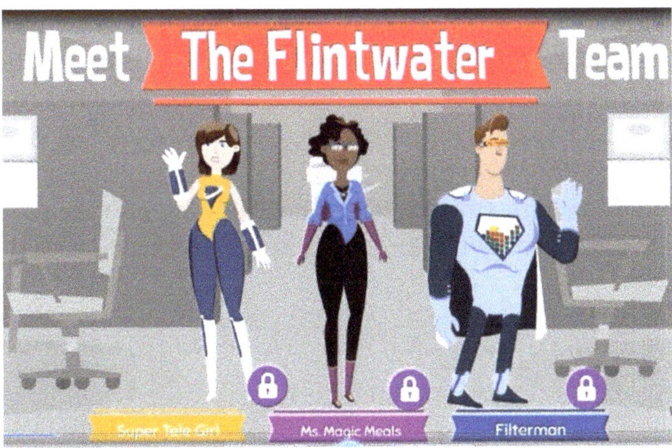

FIGURE 10.5 A team in action.

This holistic approach combines digital tools, research-based education, direct communication, goal-oriented collaboration, and creative content creation to address health concerns within the community, with a particular focus on lead poisoning and its long-term implications.

Summation

The showcase of students' assignments and applications in the context of the Community Health Outreach Program holds profound relevance in the creation of health care virtual programs. Each step of the assignment aligns with crucial aspects of developing comprehensive, community-oriented virtual initiatives. In essence, this showcase exemplifies the relevance of integrating digital tools, research-based content, direct communication, personalized goal-setting, and engaging multimedia in virtual health care initiatives. It mirrors the shift toward holistic, community-centered, and digitally driven health care practices in the evolving landscape of health care delivery.

Transformative Innovations in Health Care Informatics

The culmination of our journey in Chapter 10 unveils a tapestry of groundbreaking innovations in health care technology. Here, we witness not just conceptual ideas but tangible, real-world solutions meticulously crafted through modeling and the application of critical thinking. This segment seamlessly amalgamates cutting-edge technological leaps, positioning our students at the forefront of ushering in a new era of patient care excellence. Their endeavors showcase not only the theoretical prowess, but also the practical impact, paving the way for transformative advancements in health care.

Incorporating Smartphones for Inpatient Communication During COVID-19

A remarkable project emerging from this research highlights the indispensable role of smartphones in connecting hospital patients with their families, a need brought into sharp focus by the challenges posed during the COVID-19 pandemic. Recognizing the ubiquity of smartphones, our students ingeniously devised solutions that facilitated seamless communication—an essential element for maintaining emotional ties, especially when physical closeness was not a viable option.

Advancing Virtual Website Programs for Mental Health

These inspired minds have spearheaded the development of online platforms dedicated to addressing mental health needs. In an era when mental wellness awareness is on the rise, their initiatives provide comprehensive support and actionable steps. These digital spaces offer access to a plethora of tools, coping mechanisms, and pathways to expert guidance, marking a significant stride for individuals navigating mental health challenges.

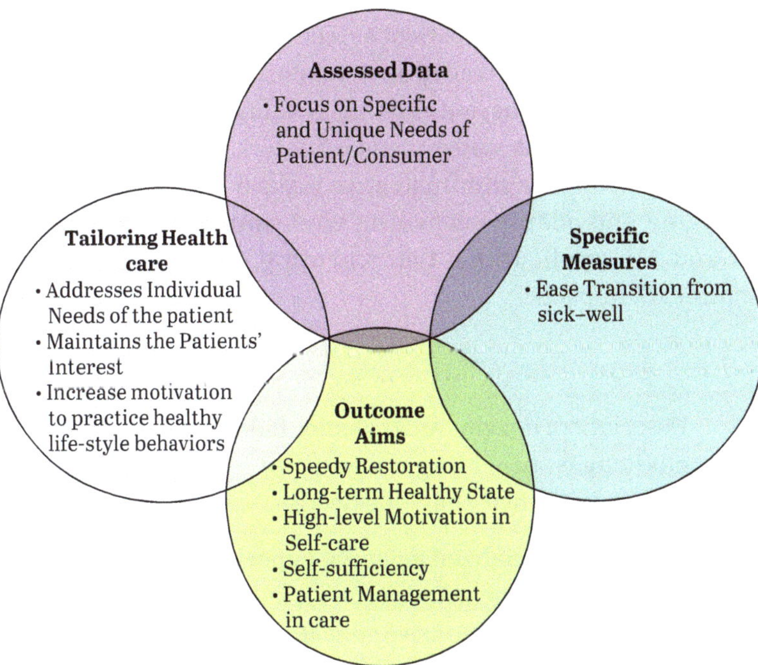

FIGURE 10.6 Tailored holistic health care.

These student-led projects exemplify the transformative shift in health care delivery, where the intersection of health care and digital innovation is strategically designed to meet people's evolving needs. By immersing themselves in contemporary challenges within HCIS, our scholars are not merely addressing the present; they are actively shaping a future when technology serves as a robust ally in health support—ensuring connectivity and delivering impactful solutions that truly matter.

Unveiling the Synergy

AI and ML Advancements in Education and Health Care Applications

AI and ML are revolutionizing the way we approach education and health care, offering innovative solutions that enhance learning experiences and improve patient outcomes. In education, AI-driven tools are reshaping traditional teaching methods, enabling personalized learning, automating grading, and providing real-time feedback to both students and educators. These advancements not only streamline administrative tasks but also foster a more engaging and adaptive learning environment. Below are key AI and ML applications transforming education and their significant impacts.

Adaptive Learning Platforms

Description: Imagine an AI mentor tailored to students' challenges, providing customized assistance that evolves with their changing needs.

Impact: Personalized learning experiences enhance student engagement and academic outcomes, fostering a dynamic and responsive educational environment.

Intelligent Tutoring Systems

Description: This strategy expedites the grading process, allowing instructors to return feedback promptly and invest more time in instructing.

Impact: Improves student comprehension, encourages independent learning, and assists educators in tailoring teaching methods to individual needs.

Automated Grading and Feedback

Description: AI assesses assignments, offers instant feedback, and highlights areas for improvement. ML monitors academic records to identify students at risk of falling behind.

Impact: Enhances efficiency in grading, provides timely feedback, and supports early interventions for struggling students.

Predictive Analytics for Student Success

Description: The fusion of AI and ML injects vitality into education by predicting student success and enabling early interventions.

Impact: Early interventions support struggling students, contributing to a higher rate of academic success.

IBM Watson for Oncology

Description: AI-powered guidance for oncologists, sifting through vast medical literature to create personalized treatment plans.

Impact: Enhances treatment precision and recommends evidence-based therapies, contributing to advancements in cancer care.

Google DeepMind's AlphaFold

Description: AI predicting protein structures with remarkable accuracy, aiding drug development and unraveling disease mysteries.

Impact: Critical for groundbreaking medical advances, especially in understanding complex diseases and developing targeted therapies.

PathAI

Description: ML expertise in analyzing pathology slides, enhancing early disease detection and accurate identification of hidden conditions.

Impact: Improves diagnostic accuracy, leading to earlier and more effective interventions.

Tempus

> Description: Utilizing ML for in-depth analysis of patient health histories and genetic information, refining individualized treatment strategies.
>
> Impact: Directs patients to suitable clinical trials, offering a significant advantage in their battle against complex illnesses.

The intertwining of AI and ML with education and health care displays the transformative potential of these technologies. As we move forward, these advancements promise not only improved learning experiences and academic outcomes but also more precise and personalized health care interventions, ultimately shaping a future when technology plays a pivotal role in enhancing human well-being.

Summary

Chapter 10 serves as the culmination of the concepts explored throughout this book, focusing on the practical application of informatics in health care and education. This chapter emphasizes the implementation of telemedicine solutions, enabling remote consultations and monitoring to enhance patient care. Additionally, it highlights the integration of e-learning platforms, making educational content more engaging and accessible.

A major component of this chapter is the development of a user-friendly telehealth platform, designed to facilitate seamless remote health care interactions while ensuring patient privacy and security. The chapter also explores the role of smart home technologies in homecare, providing essential support for daily activities and health monitoring for individuals receiving care at home.

Beyond these applications, Chapter 10 underscores the importance of innovation and creativity by promoting independent technology projects. Establishing a centralized repository for completed technological projects ensures ongoing knowledge sharing, fostering a collaborative and forward-thinking environment within organizations and institutions.

Building on the foundational knowledge from Chapters 1 through 9—including data management, interoperability, cybersecurity, and website design—this final chapter represents the transition from theory to real-world implementation. By applying informatics principles to practical scenarios, students gain hands-on experience in developing solutions that drive advancements in health care and education. Ultimately, Chapter 10 solidifies the connection between knowledge and action, equipping students with the tools to shape the future of digital health and learning.

Chapter Review Questions

Directions: Consider what you learned in this chapter as you respond to the health care scenario and questions.

Health Care Scenario: Keeping Up with the Advancements in Technology

You are tasked with implementing a telemedicine solution in a rural community with limited internet access. The goal is to improve health care access for elderly patients who have difficulty traveling to urban health care centers. How would you approach this challenge?

Multiple-Choice Questions

1. What is the first step you should take to assess the feasibility of telemedicine in this community?
    a. Conduct a survey to assess internet availability and reliability.
    b. Implement a pilot telemedicine program with a selected group of patients.
    c. Develop a detailed budget for equipment and connectivity.
    d. Design a training program for health care staff on telemedicine tools.

2. Which factor is most critical for ensuring successful telemedicine consultations in this context?
    a. High-speed internet connectivity
    b. Availability of advanced medical equipment
    c. Comprehensive patient medical history
    d. Regular maintenance of telemedicine software
3. What strategy can you employ to overcome challenges related to internet access in remote areas?
    a. Use satellite internet services.
    b. Implement a mobile telemedicine unit.
    c. Limit telemedicine to text-based consultations.
    d. Establish partnerships with local internet providers.
4. How can you ensure patient privacy and data security during telemedicine consultations?
    a. Use encryption and secure communication channels.
    b. Store patient data on local servers for quick access.
    c. Allow patients to choose their preferred communication platform.
    d. Share patient data with health care providers via email.
5. What is a potential barrier to patient acceptance of telemedicine in this community?
    a. Lack of transportation to health care facilities
    b. Concerns about the effectiveness of telemedicine
    c. Limited availability of medical specialists
    d. High costs associated with telemedicine consultations
6. Which metric should you track to evaluate the success of the telemedicine program in this community?
    a. Number of consultations conducted per month
    b. Patient satisfaction with telemedicine services
    c. Availability of health care staff for teleconsultations
    d. Cost savings compared to traditional health care visits

Answer Key

1. (a) Conduct a survey to assess internet availability and reliability.
2. (a) High-speed internet connectivity
3. (a) Use satellite internet services.
4. (a) Use encryption and secure communication channels.
5. (b) Concerns about the effectiveness of telemedicine
6. (b) Patient satisfaction with telemedicine services

Recommended Reading

Côté-Boileau, É., Denis, J. L., Callery, B., & Sabean, M. (2019). The unpredictable journeys of spreading, sustaining, and scaling health care innovations: A scoping review. *Health Research Policy and Systems, 17*, 84. https://doi.org/10.1186/s12961-019-0482-6

Pradhan, B., Bharti, D., Chakravarty, S., Ray, S. S., Voinova, V. V., Bonartsev, A. P., & Pal, K. (2021). Internet of Things and robotics in transforming current-day healthcare services. *Journal of Healthcare Engineering, 2021*, 9999504. https://doi.org/10.1155/2021/9999504

Rosser, J. C., Jr., Gentile, D. A., Hanigan, K., & Danner, O. K. (2012). The effect of video game "warm-up" on performance of laparoscopic surgery tasks. *Journal of the Society of Laparoscopic & Robotic Surgeons, 16*(1), 3–9. https://doi.org/10.4293/108680812X13291597715664

Sahal, R., Alsamhi, S. H., & Brown, K. N. (2022). Personal digital twin: A close look into the present and a step towards the future of personalized healthcare industry. *Sensors, 22*(15), 5918. https://doi.org/10.3390/s22155918

Reference

Junaid, S. B., Imam, A. A., Balogun, A. O., De Silva, L. C., Surakat, Y. A., Kumar, G., Abdulkarim, M., Shuaibu, A. N., Garba, A., Sahalu, Y., Mohammed, A., Mohammed, T. Y., Abdulkadir, B. A., Abba, A. A., Kakumi, N. A. I., & Mahamad, S. (2022). Recent advancements in emerging technologies for healthcare management systems: A survey. *Healthcare, 10*(10), 1940. https://doi.org/10.3390/healthcare10101940

Figure Credits

Fig. 10.2: Copyright © by Microsoft.

Fig. 10.3: Generated using Nawmal. Copyright © by Technologies Nawmal, Inc. Reprinted with permission.

Fig. 10.4a: Copyright © 2011 Depositphotos/svetas.

Fig. 10.4b: Copyright © 2011 Depositphotos/shopartgallery.

Fig. 10.4c: Copyright © 2019 Depositphotos/HstrongART.

Fig. 10.4d: Copyright © 2016 Depositphotos/alexraths.

Fig. 10.4e: Copyright © 2016 Depositphotos/belchonock.

Fig. 10.4f: Copyright © 2014 Depositphotos/Shebeko.

Fig. 10.4g: U.S. Food & Drug Administration, https://www.fda.gov/food/nutrition-facts-label/using-nutrition-facts-label-and-my-plate-make-healthier-choices.

Fig. 10.5a: Generated using Powtoon.com Copyright © by Powtoon.com, Inc. Reprinted with permission.

Fig. 10.5b: Generated using Nawmal. Copyright © by Technologies Nawmal, Inc. Reprinted with permission.

Glossary

Agreement on the scope of the project: A mutual understanding and definition of the project's boundaries, objectives, and deliverables.

Algorithms: Step-by-step procedures or formulas for solving problems or performing tasks, often used in computing and data analysis.

Application of processes: Utilization of established methods or procedures to achieve specific goals or outcomes.

Artificial intelligence: The simulation of human intelligence by machines, particularly computer systems capable of learning and problem solving.

Assessment of product sustainability: Evaluation of a product's ability to endure and maintain its utility over time, considering environmental, economic, and social factors.

Automated tools: Software or systems that perform tasks with minimal human intervention, often using predefined rules or algorithms.

Biometrics: Measurement and statistical analysis of people's unique physical and behavioral characteristics, used for identification and authentication.

Breach: Unauthorized access to or disclosure of sensitive or confidential information.

Business intelligence for health care: The use of data analysis tools and techniques to improve decision-making in health care organizations.

Change decision: The process of selecting and implementing a course of action to modify existing practices or procedures.

Computer system: A set of hardware components and software applications that work together to perform tasks.

Conceptualization: The process of forming abstract ideas or concepts.

Configuration: The arrangement or setup of hardware, software, or network components to achieve specific functionality.

Core concepts: Fundamental principles or key ideas central to a particular subject or discipline.

Critical thought: The objective analysis and evaluation of an issue to form a judgment.

Data: Information in raw or unorganized form that is processed to gain knowledge or insights.

Data analysis: The process of inspecting, cleansing, transforming, and modeling data with the goal of discovering useful information, conclusions, and supporting decision-making.

Data collection: The systematic gathering of data for research, analysis, or monitoring purposes.

Data elements: Individual units of information, often the smallest meaningful components of a dataset.

Data sources: Origins or locations from which data is collected or obtained.

Database breaches: Security incidents when unauthorized parties gain access to a database.

Database management: The practice of organizing, storing, and managing data in a database system.

Database schemas: Diagrams or structural representations of a database's logical or physical design.

Decision-making processes: The cognitive process of making choices or selecting a course of action among various alternatives.

Development: The process of designing, creating, and improving systems, products, or processes.

Digital applications: Software or tools designed to perform specific tasks or functions using digital technology.

Digital tools: Devices or software used for digital tasks, operations, or activities.

e-learning: Learning conducted via electronic media, typically on the internet.

Enabling: Facilitating or making possible a process, activity, or outcome.

Evaluation: The systematic assessment of the worth or significance of a particular subject, project, or program.

Fast-track methods: Accelerated approaches or strategies designed to expedite processes or projects.

Finalization of project details: The completion or conclusion of final aspects or components of a project.

Forecasting: The process of making predictions or estimates about future trends or events based on past and present data.

Hardware: Physical components of a computer system or other electronic devices.

Health: The state of being free from illness or injury.

Health care: The maintenance and improvement of physical and mental health through medical services.

Health care delivery system: The organization, financing, and provision of health care services.

Health care information systems: Systems designed to manage health care data and facilitate the delivery of health care services.

Health care organizations: Institutions or entities involved in providing health care services or managing health care systems.

Health care outcomes: The effects or results of health care interventions or treatments on patients' health.

Health care services: Medical services provided to individuals or communities to promote health and treat illness.

Health Guardian for Longevity Program: A specific program focused on promoting health and longevity.

Health informatics: The intersection of health care, information technology, and data science aimed at improving health care outcomes.

Health information: Data related to health conditions, treatments, and outcomes.

Health information systems (HIS): Information systems designed specifically for health care settings to manage health-related data.

Health information technology (HIT): Technology used to manage healthcare information and support healthcare delivery.

Health-related program: A program designed to address specific health issues or promote healthy behaviors.

Homecare: Health care services provided in a patient's home rather than in a hospital or health care facility.

Implementation: The process of putting a plan or system into effect.

Improve outcomes: To enhance or achieve better results or consequences, particularly in health care.

Informatics: The science of information, particularly the practice of information processing and management.

Information: Data that is processed and organized to convey meaning.

Information management: The systematic organization, storage, and retrieval of information.

Integrity issues: Concerns related to the accuracy, reliability, and trustworthiness of data or systems.

Interoperability: The ability of different systems or devices to exchange and interpret data.

Key challenges of the entity: Major obstacles or difficulties faced by an organization or entity.

Key principles: Fundamental beliefs, values, or rules guiding behavior or decision-making.

Knowledge management: The process of capturing, distributing, and effectively using knowledge within an organization.

Legal: Relating to laws, regulations, or legal issues.

Logic model: A visual representation of the relationship between resources, activities, outputs, outcomes, and impacts of a program or project.

Machine learning: A branch of artificial intelligence focused on developing algorithms that enable computers to learn from and make decisions or predictions based on data.

Maintenance: The process of preserving or restoring equipment, systems, or facilities to ensure continued functionality.

Management: The coordination and administration of tasks, resources, and people to achieve specific goals or objectives.

Mobile: Relating to devices or technology that is portable and typically used while on the move.

Modeling: The process of creating mathematical or computational models to simulate real-world phenomena.

Monitoring: The systematic observation, surveillance, or tracking of a process, activity, or system.

Negotiation of the contract: The process of discussing terms, conditions, and agreements to reach a mutual understanding in a contractual relationship.

Networks: Systems of interconnected computers, devices, or entities.

Optimization: The process of making something as effective or functional as possible, often involving maximizing desired outcomes or minimizing undesired ones.

Organizations: Entities or associations formed for a specific purpose, often structured with defined roles and responsibilities.

Patient care: The services and treatments provided to individuals to promote health and well-being.

Planning strategies: Methods or approaches developed to achieve goals or objectives through systematic preparation and organization.

Problem identification: The process of recognizing and defining issues or challenges that need to be addressed.

Product evaluation methods: Techniques or approaches used to assess the effectiveness, quality, or performance of a product or service.

Project details: Specific information or particulars regarding a project, including its scope, objectives, timeline, and resources.

Project management: The discipline of planning, organizing, securing, and managing resources to achieve specific goals within defined constraints.

Project scope: The extent and boundaries of what a project is supposed to accomplish, including deliverables and outcomes.

Quality improvement: Systematic efforts to enhance performance, effectiveness, and efficiency in processes, products, or services.

Rationale development: The process of establishing the reasons or justification behind a decision, action, or proposal.

Regulatory considerations: Factors or issues related to compliance with laws, rules, or regulations.

Remote monitoring: The practice of observing or supervising a system, process, or condition from a distance using technology.

Resource: Assets, materials, or capabilities used to achieve objectives or support activities.

Resource allocation: The process of distributing available resources among competing demands or needs.

Robotics: The branch of technology that deals with the design, construction, operation, and application of robots.

Role: A defined position, function, or purpose within a system, organization, or situation.

Security: Measures taken to protect against unauthorized access, use, or modification of data or systems.

Security protection frameworks: Frameworks or strategies designed to safeguard information or systems from threats or vulnerabilities.

Security systems: Systems or measures put in place to protect assets, information, or individuals from harm or unauthorized access.

Self-managers: Individuals capable of managing their own tasks, responsibilities, or health-related behaviors independently.

Software: Programs and applications that run on computer hardware to perform specific tasks or functions.

Strategic planning: The process of defining an organization's strategy or direction and making decisions on allocating resources to pursue this strategy.

Strategy: A plan of action designed to achieve a long-term or overall goal.

Structured data: Information organized in a predefined format, often in rows and columns, making it easily searchable and analyzable.

System: A set of interacting or interdependent components forming an integrated whole, often referring to software or hardware.

System selection team: A group tasked with evaluating and choosing appropriate systems or software for an organization.

Tactical planning: Short-term, specific actions and plans designed to achieve parts of a broader strategy.

Tactics: Specific actions or steps taken to accomplish a strategy or achieve specific goals.

Tangible examples pages of the website: Web pages that provide concrete instances or illustrations of concepts or content.

Target population: The specific group of individuals intended to be served or studied in a program, project, or research.

Telehealth: The use of digital communication technologies to provide healthcare services remotely.

Theories: Systematic sets of ideas intended to explain phenomena or concepts.

TIGER: Technology Informatics Guiding Education Reform, an initiative focused on integrating informatics competencies in nursing education.

Unstructured data: Information that does not have a predefined format, such as text, images, or social media posts.

Website design: The process of creating the layout, appearance, and usability of a website.

Workflow: The sequence of steps or processes through which tasks are completed in an organization or system.

Work plan: A detailed outline of tasks, timelines, and resources required to complete a project or achieve goals.

Index

T

U

V

W

About the Author

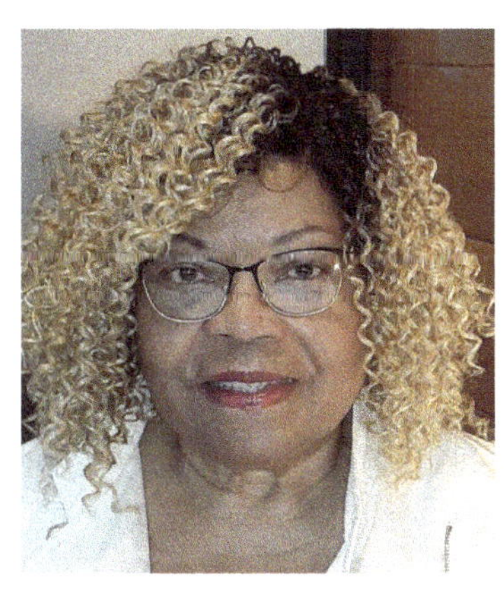

IMG 0.1

Freida Pemberton, Ed.D., Ph.D., RN-BC is a distinguished nursing professional with over five decades of expertise in nursing practice, informatics, education, research, administration, and public speaking. Her career, spanning 51 years, reflects a deep commitment to advancing healthcare and education, shaped by her personal experiences with discrimination and healthcare disparities.

As a board-certified informatics nurse for 21 years, Dr. Pemberton has significantly impacted the field through her roles as a consultant, administrator, grant reviewer, and innovator. Her work in promoting healthy lifestyle behaviors via mobile and virtual technologies exemplifies her dedication to integrating technology into healthcare.

Dr. Pemberton is a full professor of nursing at Molloy University, where she has served for 31 years. She developed the Nursing Informatics component of the Nursing Administration program and continues to advance health informatics education. She holds a Bachelor of Science in nursing from Mt. Sinai School of Nursing-City College, a master's in nursing education from New York University, an Ed.D. in curriculum and instruction from International Graduate School, and a Ph.D. in health services from Walden University.

In addition to her academic roles, Dr. Pemberton has received numerous accolades, including the Eleanor Beatrice Hull Award (June 1, 2024) from the Women's Industrial Service League for Outstanding Community Service. Her courses are highly sought after.

Dr. Pemberton's leadership extends to various school-and university-wide committees, including Faculty Council; Diversity,

Equity and Inclusion; and Graduate Policies and Planning. She has also chaired multiple committees, such as Graduate, Promotion, Distance Learning, and Middle States Student Assessment.

As an accomplished speaker and recognized expert, Dr. Pemberton has presented as the keynote speaker in Italy, Germany, Canada, West Africa, and the USA at conferences on telehealth, mobile health, and nursing informatics. She has published several articles, websites, conducted research using qualitative and quantitative designs, and developed a nonprofit 501(c)(3) public charity. She serves as an HRSA grant reviewer and editorial board member for a nursing and healthcare publication. Her work also includes leading the Global Learning for Nurses course in West Africa, integrating mobile technology to support remote client care.

Dr. Pemberton's extensive expertise in informatics and her unwavering dedication to education, healthcare, and social justice underscore her transformative impact on the profession and society at large.

www.ingramcontent.com/pod-product-compliance
Ingram Content Group UK Ltd.
Pitfield, Milton Keynes, MK11 3LW, UK
UKHW021831270726
14058UKWH00001B/92